Emotional Healing for Horses & Ponies

Stefan Ball, Heather Simpson
& Judy Howard

Emotional
Healing
for Horses
& Ponies

Index by Lyn Greenwood
Illustrated by Kate Aldous

SAFFRON WALDEN
THE C.W. DANIEL COMPANY LIMITED

First published in the United Kingdom by
The C.W. Daniel Company Limited
1 Church Path, Saffron Walden,
Essex CB10 1JP, United Kingdom

7

ISBN 978-0-85207-354-4

Designed by Jane Norman
Production in association with
Book Production Consultants plc, 25-27 High Street,
Chesterton, Cambridge CB4 1ND.

Penguin Random House is committed to a sustainable future for
our business, our readers and our planet. This book is made from
Forest Stewardship Council® certified paper.

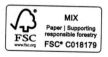

Printed and bound in Great Britain by Clays Ltd, Elcograf S.p.A.

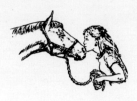

Contents

Introduction

A true story

Once there was a horse called Borane. He lived in a remote part of Europe. He was a magnificent horse, similar in appearance to Anna Sewell's *Black Beauty*.

At four years old Borane refused a water jump while taking part in one of his first competitions. To channel him towards the jump he was charged through a human tunnel that led to the edge of the water. The tunnel terrified him. As he got close to the water someone swung a rake and hit him on the rump. The prongs of the rake stuck in his tail. He clamped his tail down hard, and the handle of the rake got tangled between his legs and broke. The jagged broken end of the shaft dug into his inner thigh.

Borane was terrified. With his young female rider hanging on in fear of her life, he bolted through the water and on through the next jump, scattering and snapping wooden gates and poles. He ran for one and a half kilometres until he came to a T-junction on a busy road. Two cars swerved to miss him, and collided with each other instead. His rider flung herself to the ground, fracturing her skull and breaking her shoulder and both legs. She was unconscious for two days.

Borane's panic continued. The rake was still in his tail, the shaft still digging into his leg. He ran another kilometre or two and came to a roundabout at another busy junction. Several cars swerved to miss him. This time he slipped and fell, and at last he was caught.

Soon afterwards Borane was sold. His new owner tended his wounds and put him in a paddock with a few other horses and some cattle for company. Borane lived there for two years without much human contact. Then his owner decided it was time for him to learn to jump again and started, very gently, to school him. But the fear and terror of his last jumping experience were still with him.

Four years passed. A young girl called Claire went on holiday with her family to the area where Borane lived. Claire's mother saw Borane and bought him for her. He was shipped off to their home.

Borane was a gentle horse and loved attention. Sometimes he would wrap his head and neck around Claire to stop her leaving

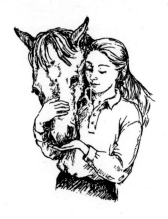

the stable. But he wasn't happy. Sometimes he seemed depressed and panicky. He had no self-confidence. One day he would overreact to situations and the next day the same things would not bother him at all. Out riding he would lose concentration. Sometimes he reacted late or became anxious and anticipated things too quickly. There were times when he was argumentative as well. Although he was loving and affectionate, he never played. Claire was concerned and worried about him.

When Claire eventually asked Borane to try jumping again he became anxious and uncooperative. He twitched and reared up, pulled away, and sometimes refused to jump at all. Occasionally he hurried through the jumps to get the whole thing over and done with. At times Claire had difficulty keeping him under control and had to leave the ring before the course was completed.

Claire's mother sought advice, and ended up seeing a complementary practitioner who made up a mixture of remedies for him to take, in water, several times daily. Two days after beginning to take his potion Borane jumped in his first competition of the season. Claire was nervous. How would Borane behave? His behaviour when they were riding and practising had been wonderful and he was like a different horse, but how would he cope under pressure in a competition?

When the day came he was excited, but there was no trace of fear and anxiety. He followed Claire's instructions to the letter and jumped beautifully. They took every fence with ease and flew round the course as if on wings. People congratulated Claire and everyone was asking what could have made such a remarkable difference to Borane.

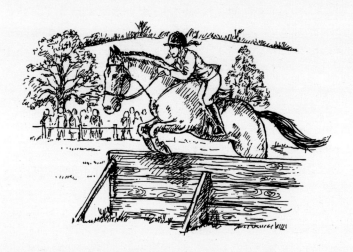

What this book can do for you

Part of the answer to their question lies in the work of a key figure in the history of 20th century medicine, Dr Edward Bach. The rest of the answer lies in the concept of *understanding*, which in this context means trying to see events from the horse's point of view. This book helps you bring these two elements together. Our aim is to help your horse attain the kind of emotional health that horses in the wild enjoy.

We start by looking at the application of Dr Bach's system of 38 flower remedies to the emotional health of horses and ponies. Part One tells you how to start thinking about your animal's individual personality and mood, how to mix remedies together, and of course when and how to give them. It lists the 38 remedies in full, tells you what each one is for, and gives examples of situations in which you could use them. If you are new to Dr Bach's work the idea of treating negative emotions with medicines might seem strange, and you might find it difficult to see how balancing emotions can affect physical problems like laminitis or strangles. These questions are addressed in Part One, and you can apply much of the information here to horses and riders alike.

Part Two is the longest section. It has two functions. The first is to provide quick access to the system when you need it. First look for the heading that most closely describes the situation that you and your horse are coping with. Then look at the suggested remedies. Once you have found one or two that seem to cover the problem re-read the full indications for those remedies as given in Part One. Cross-checking will help you select the right remedies for your horse's particular emotional state.

Part Two's second function is to deepen your knowledge of how horses think and feel. Our approach is not just ameliorative, but political. We argue that in order to have truly balanced horses we have to understand much more about what they need from their environments: social contact with other horses, the chance to form a pair-bond, and freedom from life in a cage.

Part Three provides examples of other ways to approach your horse's emotional and physical health, and suggests ways in which you can learn more about Dr Bach's work.

Trade marks

In the UK, the words 'Bach' and 'Bach flower remedies' are used as generic terms to describe the 38 remedies discovered by Dr Edward Bach. Outside the UK, 'Bach' and 'Bach Flower Remedies' are trade marks or registered trade marks and can only be used in relation to particular products from particular essence makers. The authors hereby acknowledge these and any other trade marks mentioned in the text as the property of the relevant trade mark holders.

A note on personal pronouns

Throughout the book we have tended to refer to horses as 'he' and to riders as 'she', except where the sex of the horse or rider is an important consideration. This makes it easier to say clearly who is doing what to whom. It also allows us to avoid ungrammatical ('to tell a horse's age, look at their teeth'), depersonalising ('...look at its teeth') and clumsy ('...at his or her teeth') constructions. Our use of pronouns is not meant to discriminate against male riders or female horses.

In adopting this convention we follow the lead of Mary Wanless' thoughtful book *For the Good of the Horse*.

Acknowledgements

We have had help in preparing this book. We are grateful to Lynette Mackay who allowed us to condense and reproduce some of her successful case studies. Rose Todd gave us permission to print Borane's story, which opens the introduction. Amanda Bustin of the Blue Cross allowed us to include details of the treatment given by Heather to Bud and Rosie.

Ian, Jane and Genevieve Miller at The C.W. Daniel Co. were patient beyond the call of duty with last-minute changes. Finally, and by no means least, our partners, children, friends and colleagues gave support and encouragement as usual.

If you have any ideas for improving future editions of this book or would like to tell us about your successes or failures with your horses, please write to the authors c/o The Bach Centre. The address is in Part Three.

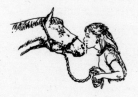

Part One

The remedies – history, description and use

Dr Bach and his discoveries

Dr Edward Bach practised medicine during the early part of the 20th century. He was a qualified surgeon who worked as a pathologist and bacteriologist, and also a well-known researcher who carried out extensive work into the relationship between chronic disease and the immune system. This culminated in the development of a group of vaccines based on different types of intestinal bacteria, which proved to be successful in combating certain chronic diseases. He was recognised around the world for this pioneering work, and enjoyed a substantial income (for the 1920s) of £5,000 a year.

Despite the success of his orthodox research Bach dreamed of finding a safer and gentler means of relieving people of their suffering. An introduction to homoeopathy gave him many of the answers he was looking for, and he began to prepare his vaccines homoeopathically. This provided a safe, minimal-dose alternative to the concentrated vaccination. It also meant that he no longer had to use injections on his patients. The homoeopathic preparations – known as nosodes – could be given by mouth, and for this reason were less intrusive and less painful.

Dr Bach was as interested in the fears and worries and hopes of his patients as he was in their physical ailments. He saw them as individuals with lives that extended beyond the bounds of the hospital ward. He would spend hours listening to what they said and taking note of their individual characters, and early on he noticed how a person's emotional outlook and attitude determined how well she would respond to treatment. The state of mind of his patients was crucial to their well-being and general state of health. Happy people did not get ill as often as unhappy people. When they did fall ill they recovered sooner.

As Bach gave the homoeopathically prepared nosodes to more and more patients he began to see how some of their personality patterns were repeated from individual to individual. People with high amounts of a particular bacteria in their intestines seemed to share the same general outlook on life. This echoed the theory in homoeopathy of the *constitutional* remedy, in other words a medicine that matched a person's type of character. To test the theory he tried predicting which nosode people would need based on their character and personality. He checked out his predictions by analysing bacteria from his patients' stomachs. The correlation between the two methods of diagnosis was so high that he eventually dispensed with clinical physical examination altogether and selected purely on the basis of emotional outlook.

Despite the success his work had achieved there were two aspects of it that he wanted to improve. First, he was using the agent of a disease – bacteria – to treat the disease, and felt that a cleaner and more wholesome approach would be to find healing plants that would have similar effects. Second – and more importantly – his nosodes treated some chronic diseases but left the general problem of illness untouched. Convinced that negative emotional outlook was what gave disease the opportunity to flourish, he saw how true healing would only come when he could find a way to treat the patient's state of mind directly. The ideal medicine would have the capacity to heal at the most fundamental level, and so prevent physical disease before it took place.

The search for these new remedies took up the rest of Bach's life. One by one he discovered 38 remedies: 36 prepared from the flowers of wild trees, shrubs and plants, one from a cultivated plant, and one from natural healing water. He finished his research in 1935, and announced that the system was complete. Just over a year later, in 1936, he died.

How flower remedies work

Each of Bach's remedies treats a specific state of mind or way of thinking. Larch is the remedy for people who lack confidence, and its action is to remove the fear of failure. Gentian gives encouragement to those who have suffered a set-back. Clematis is for when we daydream and find it hard to concentrate on the present. Most of the time we feel a mix of emotions, so we can combine individual remedies together to create a personal blend. Hundreds of millions of combinations are possible. This flexibility means that 38 remedies can treat the varied emotional needs of every living thing, making Dr Bach's system unique in its combination of power and simplicity. But how exactly does the system do what it claims to do?

One way to explain how the remedies work is to think of emotional states as vibrations or sound waves. A pure note rings clear, and reflects a positive, healthy emotion such as love, kindness or joy. The sound of a cracked or muffled note is repressed and distorted, negative and unhealthy – the equivalent of hate, cruelty or despair. The 38 remedies vibrate at the same pitch as the basic positive emotions. A correctly selected remedy resonates with the repressed emotion and helps it ring out clearly and strongly once more. The note sings and the negative distortion disappears.

This description is not very 'scientific' but it is a helpful metaphor for energies that science is only beginning to explore. In Dr Bach's day the link between positive emotions and health was just as vague and unscientific, but solid research now supports the relationship, and molecular messengers between emotional states and the immune system have been identified and named. Psychoneuroimmunology – the study of the way the central nervous and immune systems interact – has shown that happiness and positive emotions really do affect physical health, just as Dr Bach claimed. We can only guess what remarkable rediscoveries science will make in the future.

The 38 remedies

When you buy Bach flower remedies in a shop you will see that they are numbered from 1 to 38 according to their alphabetical order in English. We have listed them in this same order so that you can look them up more easily when you are using Part Two of this book.

Remember that Bach remedies rebalance emotions, which in turn helps the body to find its own natural state of health. The remedies do not have a direct effect on physical problems or symptoms. You should always consult a vet if you think your horse is in pain or needs medical attention.

One of the main uses for remedies when dealing with horses is to help them recover from the stress of living with people. If you want to start selecting remedies for your horse at once we strongly recommend that you read at least Parts One and Two of this book before doing so. This will help you avoid misunderstanding the emotional causes of your horse's behaviour and so selecting the wrong remedies. Incorrectly selected remedies will do no harm, but they will not help the situation improve.

1. Agrimony

General indication – used to help those who hide their troubles behind a cheerful face.

Horses of this nature may be difficult to identify because you often have to guess at the torture concealed inside an apparently cheerful animal. They will be inclined to be good-natured, happy, peace-loving creatures who try to defuse painful situations or potential confrontations, perhaps by turning them into a game. Agrimony horses may be restless when you would expect them to rest, or seem vaguely agitated yet remain playful and in good humour. They are especially fond of company and activity because it helps them take their minds off their worries.

Things to look for:

- ∩ horses who are particularly playful when under stress, or when there is emotional discord in the stable (see page 101 for more examples of displacement behaviour);

- ∩ obvious injury or illness accompanied by playful behaviour;

- ∩ restlessness and sleeplessness – but remember that the average horse only dozes in snatches of four or five minutes at a time at any time of the day and night, and only sleeps about three hours in total, so don't assume sleeplessness without real cause.

Jake

Jake would scratch and paw at the ground when he was left alone. He was never quiet, and his rider repeatedly found herself reassuring him that there was nothing to be scared of. After a few remedies had been tried without success he was given Agrimony for the inner torture that he was trying to displace by pawing in the stable.

After just one day he was able to stay by himself without fretting, and he started to gain weight as his appetite improved.

Note: *Long-term solutions to this kind of problem involve real changes in management routines. See page 101 for displacement behaviour; and page 150 for how to help horses confined to stables.*

2. Aspen

General indication – used to treat vague, nameless fears, and feelings of uneasiness and foreboding without there being anything specific to feel anxious about.

Horses in need of Aspen will seem afraid of something that is not really there. Theirs is a free-floating anxiety, not attached to anything specific like a loud noise or strangers, but simply in the air. Remember however that the fact that *you* can't identify the reason for a horse's anxiety does not prove that the horse doesn't know what he is scared of. In practice it is usually a good idea to try the remedy for a known fear – Mimulus – before turning to Aspen.

Things to look for:

- ∩ horses who seem nervous and anxious in familiar, safe environments;

- ∩ horses who jump and run at every sound, even when the cause of the sound is known to be non-threatening;

- ∩ sudden, unexplained panic, perhaps with rolling eyes and sweating.

3. Beech

General indication – given to encourage the latent sense of tolerance and understanding in those who are critical and intolerant of other ways of life. Those needing this remedy will believe that their own way of doing things is the only sensible and reasonable one, and that everyone who does things differently is simply stupid.

Horses in a Beech state may refuse to eat if you don't give them their usual food. They become irritable quite quickly, and will take the time to let you know of their disapproval.

Things to look for:

∩ horses who behave irritably when their normal living arrangements are disrupted;

∩ horses who show intolerance of new people, foods, animals, etc.;

∩ horses who overreact to minor irritations such as brushing through long grass;

∩ horses who protest vocally or kick or move about when you try to groom or saddle them.

Note: *Problems with saddling or taking the bit are often caused by pain. Always check with the vet before assuming they are due to a Beech state.*

4. Centaury

General indication – used to encourage the will-power of those who are easily dominated. Those needing Centaury will do anything for anyone, and are always obliging and ready to serve, but can find it hard to say 'no' and at the extreme fail to live their own lives at all.

Horses of this type are soft and compliant. They don't tend to fight back if they are subject to aggression or attack. They may be quiet and introverted and go out of their way to help another creature. Other animals and riders will find it easy to dominate them.

Things to look for:

- horses who are bullied by other horses and can't seem to respond or escape;

- horses in a herd who seem not to be getting their fair share of food or shelter;

- 'soppy' horses who will do anything for you but seem lost when you are not there;

- horses who have trouble setting sensible boundaries to their personal space;

- horses who never take the initiative and always wait to be led.

5. Cerato

General indications – used to strengthen the self-belief of those who do not trust their own instincts. Cerato creatures tend to question their decisions as soon as they have made them. They seek the reassurance of others, hoping for confirmation that they are doing the right thing, and may accept bad advice and so end up doing the wrong thing.

The typical Cerato indications of hesitancy and mimicry can both be normal behaviour in horses. Copying others, for example, is a perfectly natural part of play. But genuine Cerato horses will look for approval before doing anything at all. Even after the event they may look for confirmation that they have acted correctly or appropriately.

Things to look for:

- horses who seem to need more reassurance than others;

- horses who copy other horses more readily than most, and so behave out of character.

6. Cherry Plum

General indications – given to help bring calm and restore sanity to those who feel on the point of losing control, and perhaps committing some violence that they would never consider while in their right minds.

Cherry Plum is a fear remedy. Just as children are frightened by their own temper tantrums, so horses can be made hysterical

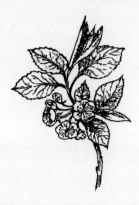

and terrified when their frustration gets the better of them. Cherry Plum is the remedy to maintain and restore self-possession and remove this kind of fear.

Things to look for:

∩ horses who injure themselves, for example biting their flanks or throwing themselves around the stable, especially when the behaviour seems compulsive or manic;

∩ horses who panic and do anything to escape, regardless of the risk of injuring themselves;

∩ horses who strike out with their forelegs or bite, and then immediately seem frightened at what they have done;

∩ uncontrolled attacks on smaller animals or other horses.

7. Chestnut Bud

General indications – used to help those who repeat the same mistakes and do not seem to learn from their errors or from watching the example of others.

This remedy can be given to horses who take a long time to learn how life with humans and other horses can be made to work. But it isn't a panacea for any horse who does not do exactly what you want. There may be very good reasons why your horse is not learning from you, and if you are the one making mistakes you might think about taking Chestnut Bud yourself.

Things to look for:

- ∩ horses who can't learn simple rules and moves despite repeated (and gentle) encouragement;

- ∩ horses who repeat behaviour despite the bad effects that follow, such as the colt who continues to make overtures to an adult mare despite the fact that he always receives a kick for his trouble.

8. Chicory

General indications – used to bring out the positive, generous side of loving individuals who need to be loved in return, and who get upset if they don't get the attention they feel they deserve. Chicory types at their most negative are possessive and emotionally manipulative.

Horses of this type are happiest when they are able to show and receive affection. They may be unwilling to share you and so seem possessive when other people or animals are around. They may pine for you when you are not there.

You may also see Chicory states develop between horses. But be aware of our natural tendency to imagine that horses are just like human beings. Behaviour that looks like Chicory to us may be neutral in a herd animal, and simply reflect his need to be part of the herd, or the strong drive he has to pair up with another horse for increased safety and mutual support (see page 75).

Things to look for:

∩ horses who seek attention from 'their' human but show little liking for strangers;

∩ horses who guard and shepherd another horse to an excessive degree;

∩ horses who compete for your attention, either with your other horses, or when you talk to other riders, etc.

Chicory is sometimes thought of as the 'controlling mother' or 'mother-in-law' remedy, despite the fact that a Chicory human is just as likely to be male. In equine society the stereotype is reversed, and stallions chivvying their herds along and rounding up stray members of their harem are more obvious Chicory examples than the average mare.

9. Clematis

General indications – used to help ground those who live in dreams of future happiness. The remedy helps them act in the present and make happiness come true now.

Clematis horses seem to fall into a drowse more easily and more often than other horses. They have little liking for or link with everyday reality, and instead live in a world of their own, not paying attention to what is going on around them any more than they absolutely have to. (NB: typical Clematis type indications could be symptoms of ill health. Always ask the vet to check your horse if he seems sleepy or inattentive.)

Things to look for:

- ∩ excessive sleepiness;

- ∩ horses who get into accidents through not paying attention to where they are;

- ∩ horses who do not notice positive stimuli such as the approach of a pair-bond or the arrival of food.

10. Crab Apple

General indications – given to help those who feel ashamed or disgusted at their own appearance, or who feel contaminated, whether by disease, poison or unclean living. Crab Apple types tend to fuss over minor details, particularly those related to cleanliness, and have a tendency towards trivial obsessions and compulsive behaviour.

Horses in this state may appear particularly distressed when suffering from skin complaints or parasite infestation. They may exhibit compulsive behaviour, and be especially fussy about their living arrangements.

Things to look for:

- ∩ horses who are overly fastidious, for example refusing to graze in areas that other horses are happy to accept;

- ∩ horses who exhibit stereotypical behaviour, such as weaving and wind-sucking (see page 106);

- ∩ horses who seem depressed due to parasitic infestation, bowel problems, etc.;

- ∩ depression linked with any problem that affects the way the horse looks.

11. Elm

General indications – used to restore a sense of self-assurance to those who have accepted too much responsibility and as a result are suffering from a temporary loss of confidence. In contrast with the Larch state (see page 33) Elm types know they can do things, but sometimes feel overwhelmed by the sheer number or scale of the things they have to do.

Your normally capable and self-confident horse may seem dejected and down in the mouth when he is in an Elm state. This usually happens when the Elm horse has something new to deal with on top of an already full workload.

Things to look for:

∩ horses who are struggling to cope with additional pressures or demands, such as the birth of a foal or a change of routine;

∩ capable horses who lose their confidence when they are ill.

12. Gentian

General indications – given to those who have suffered a set-back of some kind and as a result feel discouraged and despondent. The Gentian state is a mild form of depression, and the remedy gives encouragement so that it can be overcome quickly.

Try Gentian whenever something has gone wrong in your horse's life and he responds by losing heart. The cause of the problem could be anything from missing out on a regular treat to the onset of a serious and painful medical problem like laminitis.

Things to look for:

∩ horses who respond to set-backs by withdrawing or becoming despondent;

∩ horses who seem inclined to give up easily when they fall ill.

13. Gorse

General indications – this remedy is given to those who have gone a step beyond the Gentian state, and really have given up. It may be obvious to everyone else what the solution to a problem is, but those in the Gorse state decide that nothing more can be done and stop looking for answers. If they do seek solutions it is usually at the prompting of someone else. Their attitude to every effort is a pessimistic conviction of failure.

Horses in this state are very down and seem full of despair. They make no effort to enjoy life or recover from illness. The remedy helps strengthen their natural hope and faith so that they can fight illness more effectively.

Things to look for:

- ♫ horses who react very badly when things go wrong, and do not respond easily to encouragement from you;

- ♫ Gentian horses (see above) who have fallen further down into despair;

- ♫ horses who have stopped fighting illness and do not try to get better.

14. Heather

General indications – used to widen the perspective of those who are overly wrapped up in their own lives. Those in a negative Heather state can't bear to be alone and will seek attention from anyone. They enjoy talking about their troubles. They latch on to willing listeners and make it difficult for them to get away. The remedy encourages Heather types to understand the needs of others and allows them to see their own problems in perspective.

Heather horses will attach themselves to anyone who is prepared to give them even the minimum of encouragement.

They may show no real preference for their pair-bond horse or rider, or for anyone else. Any audience will do as long as it is prepared to put up with their demand for company and constant attention.

Things to look for:

- ∩ horses who like people and other horses around, including strangers, and demand attention from them, sometimes using inappropriate behaviour to get what they want;

- ∩ horses who are very vocal or demonstrative and insist on being heard;

- ∩ horses who try to keep with you as much as possible, but do not respond to your calls or signals.

There is a good example of a Heather state in the story of Bud on page 126.

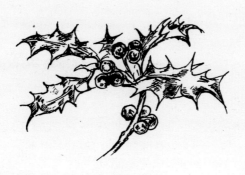

15. Holly

General indications – given to encourage the hidden loving heart of those who give way to strong negative feelings about others, such as hatred, suspicion, envy or spite.

Wrongly thought of as being the 'remedy for anger' – there are in fact many possible remedies for anger – Holly is often given to aggressive horses inappropriately, to such an extent that some people treating animals prefer not to use this remedy at all. It may be indicated if your horse is especially suspicious of people's motives or jealous of a newcomer to the stable, but if for example there are symptoms of fear then Mimulus (see page 34) or Rock Rose (see page 41) would be preferred. Horses are prey animals and humans are predators, so in the equine world fear of humans is far more likely than hatred and spite.

Things to look for:

- attacks or aggression towards another horse, where the attacks seem designed to hurt rather than intimidate;

- aggressive body language and threats towards others (but only where you have ruled out more likely causes, such as fear or play behaviour);

- attacks on potential rivals, such as newly acquired horses and ponies.

In his book *The Man Who Listens to Horses* the US horse whisperer Monty Roberts tells the story of In Tissar, a stallion who attacked mares and people and seemed to show psychotic and sadistic tendencies. On the face of it this would seem to be a classic Holly horse. However, the key to selecting remedies for a problem like this would be to look for the underlying cause. Even if we did decide to select Holly for the horse's immediate desire to hurt we would still want to look further to see what pressures had left him in this extreme state and select further remedies on that basis. The lives of stallions are often hideously traumatic and always benefit from further investigation. (see page 76).

16. Honeysuckle

General indications – given to help those who live in the past, either reliving past happiness or wallowing in regrets and sad

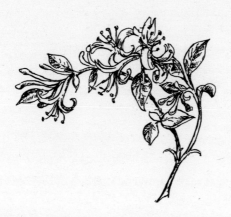

recollections. Honeysuckle helps them enjoy the present more, and renews faith that there is always something in life worth looking forward to.

Signs of a Honeysuckle state in a horse include a lack of interest in what is going on today, and a liking for places or activities that he associates with the past or with previous owners or pair-bonds. Grieving horses who have lost beloved companions might need this remedy if the grieving process goes on longer than normal (see page 130 for more on grief and parting).

Things to look for:

- ∩ dreaminess and inattention (see also Clematis);
- ∩ horses who pull towards former homes or routes associated with former owners;
- ∩ failure to thrive in new situations;
- ∩ homesickness and pining.

17. **Hornbeam**

General indications – used to give a boost to those who find it difficult to get started, or who feel tired at the mere thought of the tasks ahead. For this reason Hornbeam is often described as the 'Monday morning remedy'.

Look for listlessness and a lack of energy in horses who have rested well and should by rights be full of life. As in all such cases obtain the advice of a vet first in order to ensure that there is no organic reason for the unexplained tiredness.

Things to look for:

- Ω tiredness that seems to wear off as the day goes on;

- Ω horses who are reluctant to exercise but full of energy once they begin;

- Ω reluctance to begin an everyday activity – for example, horses who sniff at their food, and go away and return several times before starting to eat.

18. **Impatiens**

General indications – given to bring calm and patience to those who live life in a rush, or who are agitated or irritable when things go wrong or there is a delay.

Horses in need of Impatiens will always want to be getting on to the next thing, even when the current thing is something they like or are interested in. They may behave especially badly if they are forced to wait for food or exercise or if there is any other delay in their daily routine.

Things to look for:

- Ω horses who rush around a lot and are never still;

- Ω horses who go from one activity to another very quickly;

- ∩ reluctance to stay with the herd or with other, slower or less decisive animals;

- ∩ frequent mishaps and minor accidents, caused by not taking sufficient time before taking action;

- ∩ irritability that comes and goes quickly.

Rendezvous

A 12-year-old called Rendezvous was put into temporary training. Generally she was a sweet-natured mare with a fairly stable character. But when she arrived at the stables she was worried and nervous about her new surroundings. And above all she was extremely impatient. When ridden, she could hardly bear to wait for the rider to mount, and would get very upset if she was asked to stop for any reason after work had begun. She was always in a rush, and became extremely frustrated when held back from where she wanted to go.

Three remedies were given in all, including Impatiens. Within three days Rendezvous was calm, relaxed and affectionate. She would wait quietly for the rider to mount or take off the exercise rug.

Note: *Many other remedies would have been considered in this case, including Star of Bethlehem, Walnut and Mimulus. See page 164 for tips on introducing horses to new yards successfully and with the minimum of trauma.*

19. Larch

General indications – used as a treatment for lack of confidence in those who think they are not good enough and so are bound to fail. This becomes an excuse – sometimes a welcome excuse – not to try things in the first place, or to stop trying at the first set-back.

Look for any avoidance of challenges, whether the challenge comes from other horses or from the environment, and a generally unadventurous approach to life. Larch can also be used whenever a horse is facing a particularly difficult task, such as learning to jump or integrating with a new herd, and seems to lack the essential self-belief needed to make a success of it.

Things to look for:

ᴖ horses who avoid more dominant horses, noisy dogs, friendly strangers, etc. (see also Mimulus);

ᴖ horses who are hesitant faced with new situations, foods or environments;

ᴖ horses who tend to rely on others to make the first move in any encounter.

Blade

Blade was a show jumper. He became extremely nervous and anxious when asked to learn something new, and seemed to expect to fail. He also became more and more stressed the longer he had to stay in the arena.

Blade was given several remedies, including Mimulus to help with his fear of new situations and of having to perform in front of a crowd, and Larch to help him believe in his ability to do things well.

As a result Blade was a lot calmer in the arena. He would still get a little wound up, but never to such an extent that he and his rider could not control what was happening.

(See page 165 for more on helping competitor horses.)

20. Mimulus

General indications – this is given to those who feel fearful or anxious about something specific. The 'something' can be tangible, such as a particular person or type of animal, or it can be

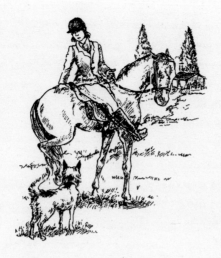

something abstract, such as illness or hunger – but in all cases it is something that can be named. Mimulus is also used to help those who tend to be shy and timid, and so find it difficult to interact with others.

The horse in need of Mimulus may appear timid and withdrawn, similar to a Larch or Centaury horse. He may start violently at loud noises and show obvious signs of fear in the presence of whatever it is that he is afraid of.

Things to look for:

- ∩ fearful body language, such as head shying and wide or rolling eyes;

- ∩ fear-based aggression, such as rearing up and kicking out with the hind feet;

- ∩ attempts to avoid specific people or situations, such as the farrier or having to get into a horse trailer;

- ∩ horses who start when there is an unexpected noise;

- ∩ reluctance to approach strangers, other horses, etc.

First Freedom

First Freedom was a six-year-old stallion who was competing at quite a high level. He was a genuine, sweet-natured horse, but he became really stressed when he had to work. He could be going along quite calmly when he would suddenly blow up and take off as if something were going to get him from behind. When practising piaffing – moving at a high, slow, trotting pace – he would lather up with fear.

Several remedies were prescribed, among them Mimulus for what seemed to be a known fear – i.e. the fear of being caught by a tiger. Within 24 hours there was a huge improvement. First Freedom went through piaffe training calmly, and for the very first time was quiet enough to practise passage. He was consistently on the bit instead of being high, low and all over the place. There was no sweat, no straining tendons, no bulging eyes – a really remarkable change.

Wendy Pride

Wendy Pride was a young mare. She had been backed then left unridden for a year before going into training, and she was nervous under saddle. She tended to run away when ridden and found everything new and strange. Otherwise her temperament was good. She seemed quiet, gentle and approachable, and enjoyed human company.

Again the main remedy for Wendy Pride was Mimulus, to deal with the fear of being ridden and the fear of new experiences. After taking the remedies for some time she was much more confident under saddle.

21. Mustard

General indications – given to help those who feel unhappy and gloomy, as if their lives were blighted, but who can think of nothing that would justify this feeling. Often all is well and they should be happy, yet still they feel full of deep melancholy and unhappiness.

Look for obvious signs of depression in a horse whose present conditions – turned out with a settled pair-bond, well fed and with room to stretch his legs – do not seem to justify the way he feels. (Always get an opinion from the vet in cases of sudden, unexplained switches of mood, as these can indicate the presence of organic disease.)

Things to look for:

- ∩ gloom that descends out of the blue, when all environmental conditions seem right;
- ∩ depressed body language or posture.

22. Oak

General indications – used to help those steady and reliable types who assume that their great strength has no limits. They are capable of amazing feats of endurance, but continue long after they should have rested and in the end may crack under the strain.

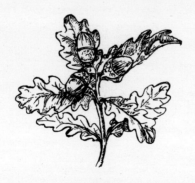

The remedy has a twofold action: restoring expended will-power and determination, and teaching restraint and the ability to stop without being broken first.

Oak-type horses are methodical rather than vivacious, more plodders than racers. Their strength is in stamina and reliability. They do not complain even under extreme pressure, but at difficult times you can give them the remedy to help them take better care of themselves. Boxer, the draught horse in George Orwell's *Animal Farm*, was a typical Oak horse. His response to every disaster and failure was to work harder, until in the end he collapsed in the shafts of his cart while trying to move yet another huge load of stone.

Things to look for:

∩ strong, reliable, steady plodders who have a sudden breakdown in health;

∩ horses who try to struggle through their normal routine despite illness and exhaustion.

23. Olive

General indications – this remedy helps restore those who feel exhausted after making some great effort – whether mental, spiritual or physical. It is often contrasted with Hornbeam (see page 32), which is for tiredness before any effort has been made.

Olive can be used to help horses who are recovering from illness and are exhausted by the process of convalescence.

Things to look for:

∩ exhaustion after a period of activity;

∩ fatigue caused by a struggle against illness or disease.

Rubino

Rubino was a very likeable character. He tried hard to please and was very affectionate, always ready for a pat and a cuddle. He had been away at a veterinary clinic for about ten days. When he came back he was skinny, and he looked really down and dejected. He had no energy at all under saddle and after ten minutes he was sweating so much that he was lathering. He was physically unable to trot out. After nearly a week in this state he was given Olive for the physical and mental exhaustion caused by his treatment at the vet's.

After three or four days there was an improvement, and Rubino didn't seem to find his training so hard. After six days he was alive again, and the old sparkle was back in his eye.

24. Pine

General indications – given to those who feel guilt about things done or left undone. Even if they have not committed any wrong action they will take the blame, sometimes excusing the real guilty party in the process.

It's easy to give Pine to horses in error. If your horse has done something 'wrong' such as escaping from his field you may get angry. The horse may lower his head towards the ground to show submission and appease your anger. You think he is 'looking guilty' and select Pine, but the horse may not think he has done anything wrong at all, and if he doesn't then Pine will do him no good.

A genuine Pine state can be hard to spot in animals as generally morose and edgy behaviour may be the only evidence you have. You will have to rely on some intelligent guesswork based on your own instincts and a careful assessment of the situation.

Things to look for:

∩ submissive behaviour when the horse has done something 'wrong', or when something has gone wrong generally – but examine your own behaviour first, and consider other remedies instead of Pine.

25. Red Chestnut

General indications – used to help restore calm and clear-thinking to those who are overanxious about the well-being of loved ones. They fear something terrible will happen to those they care about.

 One sign that this remedy is needed may be overaggressiveness by a dam towards anyone who tries to get near her foal. This is a natural response, but where the concern is exaggerated try Red Chestnut to restore a sense of proportion. (Chicory could also be helpful – see page 24.)

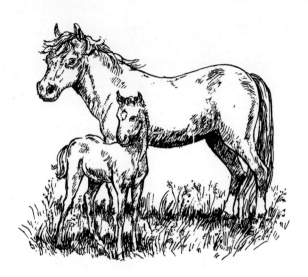

Things to look for:

 ∩ a mare who displays fear or fear aggression when anyone approaches her foal;

 ∩ horses who become especially anxious when their foal or pair-bond – or you – is out of sight;

 ∩ horses who look out anxiously for the return of their pair-bond or human carer.

26. Rock Rose

General indications – used to comfort those who are in the grip of absolute terror, either at something that is happening to them, or at the sight of something happening to another creature.

In practice it can be difficult to draw a firm line between the horse who needs Mimulus and the one who needs Rock Rose. The key lies in the intensity of the fear: in the Rock Rose state the horse will be terrified and panic-stricken. He may go berserk with fear if he can't get away and attack everything (in which case Cherry Plum has a part to play as well).

Things to look for:

∩ panic – the horse may sweat profusely and shake with fear;

∩ horses whose fear is so great that they freeze and can't act at all;

∩ desperate attempts to escape;

∩ desperate attack when escape isn't possible.

27. Rock Water

General indications – given to encourage mental and emotional flexibility in those who drive themselves hard. Rock Water types set themselves high targets and gain satisfaction and pleasure from self-denial. They start out with the idea that the end justifies the means – they must suffer in order to achieve perfection – but discipline and self-abnegation quickly become ends in themselves.

The Rock Water horse may appear driven to carry out his 'duties', and be keen to take part in relatively boring (for him) activities such as schooling even when he is tired or ill. He may live in a very regimented way, always performing the same actions at the same time and getting upset if he is obliged to break his routine. (See page 96 for more insight into the normal attitudes of horses towards routine.)

Things to look for:

   ∩ excessive dislike of changes to an established routine;

   ∩ regular habits continued despite illness and bad weather.

28. Scleranthus

General indications – used to encourage decisiveness in those who are unable to choose between the options in front of them.

A horse who needs Scleranthus will appear indecisive, sometimes even in trivial matters such as choosing which corner of a field to stand in. Scleranthus is also associated with mood swings and generalised emotional imbalance, and with other forms of imbalance such as dizziness and travel sickness. Remember though that you should always consult a vet to rule out possible organic causes for physical symptoms.

Things to look for:

   ∩ horses who hesitate when faced with decisions;

   ∩ horses who go from one thing to another and back again, without really settling;

   ∩ frequent mood swings;

   ∩ dizziness and frequent falls;

   ∩ 'travel sickness' – the design of their palates means horses can't vomit in the same way we do, but they can still feel nauseous and in extreme cases may expel the contents of their stomachs out through their nostrils.

29. Star of Bethlehem

General indications – this remedy gives comfort to those suffering from a shock of some kind, and to those who feel great loss following a sudden bereavement.

Star of Bethlehem is often given to horses rescued from mistreatment or cruelty, and as such it is a popular stand-by treatment in many animal shelters and rescue homes.

Things to look for:

- ∩ horses (especially from rescue homes) who seem to have difficulty adjusting to kind treatment;

- ∩ evidence of past or present mistreatment or trauma;

- ∩ deaths or departures in the close equine or human family;

- ∩ unaccountable changes of character or behaviour following a shock.

Shadow

Shadow was a small white pony owned by a child. He was eight years old and was used for general riding. A quiet little pony with a gentle nature, he was interested in what was going on but at the same time a little reserved. He was extremely head shy, but only with adults. If an adult approached him in a hurry he would panic and his head would go up, but children could do what they wanted and he was fine.

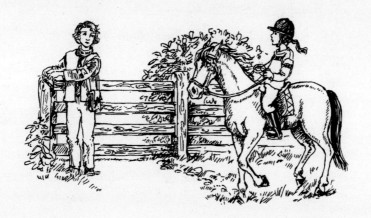

Selection was by guesswork, for nothing was known about Shadow's past or his previous owners. But on the assumption that something must have happened – it is not usual for a horse to be head shy for no reason – Star of Bethlehem was selected for past trauma, plus Mimulus for his apparent fear of being mistreated around the head.

Results were excellent. Shadow did not entirely lose his anxiety about adults, but he was no longer head shy and didn't show the same amount of fear.

30. Sweet Chestnut

General indications – given to encourage those who are suffering from complete and utter anguish and despair. The Sweet Chestnut state comes at the end of the road, where everything is bleak and not even death offers a way out.

This remedy is often used along with Star of Bethlehem for horses who have given up on life after the death of a beloved human or equine companion. It can also be used for very ill animals who appear to be in great anguish.

Things to look for:

- genuine and deep suffering;
- grave or terminal illness;
- horses who seem to have lost all hope, where you yourself can see no solution;
- inconsolable grief.

31. Vervain

General indications – used to give more balance and poise to those who are overfull of life and commitment. Sometimes enthusiasm goes too far and leads to fanaticism or emotional and physical burn-out, and Vervain is the remedy when this state of imbalance threatens.

Vervain horses are interested and enthusiastic about things. They come running up as soon as you come into the field, wanting to greet you and find out what is going to be happening today. At the same time they have a strong sense of right and wrong, and if they feel you have been too rough with them they will be quick to protest.

Things to look for:

∩ overexuberance and overenthusiasm;

∩ hyperactivity (see page 108);

∩ fiery anger at injustice;

∩ horses who get frustrated quickly when illness, confinement or incapacity mean that they can't go about their normal affairs.

Don

Don was a seven-year-old gelding. He suffered from chronic eczema. No matter how much he was brushed, old skin continued to flake off and lie through his coat, so that he looked in really poor condition. His personality was generally stressed and tense. He never stood still for a second, and was always licking and chewing with his mouth and lips. He was eager under saddle and unable to slow down.

The main remedy chosen for Don was Vervain to help him to take things a little easier. Vervain was preferred to Impatiens – another possibility – because he was eager to get involved rather than just wanting to get things finished quickly.

Within a week of using the remedies Don's coat and character both improved. The dandruff disappeared and he seemed calmer and happier.

32. Vine

General indications – this remedy is used to encourage the positive side of leadership in those who sometimes use force to get what they want. Vine types know their own minds and want others to do things their way. In a negative state they don't care much how they achieve this.

The Vine horse is the true dominant, and in the wild would be challenging for a position as stallion or alpha mare in a herd. The remedy encourages a gentler side to the qualities of determination and strength, so that the horse can assume his rightful place without feeling the need to demonstrate his power all the time. (See page 73 for more on dominance behaviour among horses.)

Things to look for:

∩ bullying of other horses;

∩ pinning back ears and chasing other horses, or head- snaking;

∩ other forms of physical threat and intimidation.

33. Walnut

General indications – given to those who are being led astray by outside influences, past or present, and to those who are going through a time of change and need help to adjust.

Sometimes Walnut is given to horses who are having trouble being themselves because of the influence of other, more dominant horses – although Centaury (see page 21) may be a better choice in many cases. Otherwise, the commonest use for Walnut is when a change in the horse's universe has had an unsettling effect. Moving to a new yard, having to assimilate into an existing herd, a change of owner or rider – all these situations suggest Walnut as a likely remedy.

Things to look for:

- ∩ horses who need help adjusting to changes such as moving or the arrival of new companions;

- ∩ horses struggling to cope with life changes, such as weaning, teething, pregnancy, disability, or infirmity in old age;

- ∩ a horse who comes under the influence of other horses or is disturbed by dogs, children or other outside influences.

34. Water Violet

General indications – sometimes self-reliance and a liking for one's own company can build up barriers to the rest of creation, leaving one isolated and unable to make contact with others. Water Violet is the remedy to help soften those in this state so that they can take the steps necessary to help the barriers come down.

True loners are rare in the horse world, as the horse is a social animal who needs company to survive in the wild. Spotting a Water Violet horse involves comparing his behaviour against norms for the average horse. Water Violet horses are not shy or fearful like Mimulus horses, but simply prefer to be by themselves more than most, or show a marked preference for being alone with their pair-bond and away from the rest of the herd. The Water Violet remedy helps when horses like this need to get along with the wider world but no longer know how.

Things to look for:

- ∩ horses who are aloof and reject familiarity, but show no sign of fear;

- ∩ relative loners who prefer to keep to themselves, or choose their companions with special care.

35. White Chestnut

General indications – used to still worrying, repetitive thoughts and mental arguments.

In this state horses may appear distracted, agitated or inattentive. Something in their lives is bothering them and stopping them from concentrating on what they are doing.

Things to look for:

∩ restlessness;

∩ inability to concentrate or to enjoy quiet moments.

36. Wild Oat

General indications – this remedy is given to those who want to do something worthwhile with their lives but don't know what that something should be. They feel frustrated at their lack of commitment and purpose, and may drift through lack of direction.

In the case of horses, this remedy state is difficult to spot, so you are relying a lot on your intuition. Wild Oat can be useful – used along with Walnut – when an activity that was once enjoyed is now no longer possible, so that the horse is left without an aim in life. This could happen to a horse who has always lived an active life as a hunter, and now through old age or incapacity has to adjust to retirement, and feels frustrated and unsatisfied with everything. Taking Wild Oat may help him to focus better and find new reasons to live.

Things to look for:

∩ aimless behaviour;

∩ inability to settle into a lifestyle.

37. Wild Rose

General indications – given to those who resign themselves without struggling to whatever life throws their way. In a positive state they are happy-go-lucky and relaxed but when out of balance they feel that life is passing them by.

Wild Rose horses do not get very enthusiastic or upset about anything. If they could talk they would be saying 'So what?', even in situations that other horses would find exciting.

Things to look for:

∩ lack of interest in the good things in life;

∩ acceptance of grooming, turn-out, etc. but without enthusiasm;

∩ horses who are fit and well but lack energy and motivation.

Note: *Lack of interest can also be a first sign of illness, so ask the vet to check your horse over if he displays these symptoms.*

38. Willow

General indications – used to encourage a more positive, generous outlook in those who blame others for their troubles and sink into grumbling resentment and self-pity.

Willow can be difficult to spot in horses because there are always alternative remedies such as Wild Rose and Gentian that might apply. In general, Willow horses tend to be introverted and seem introspective. This is often the case with cold-blooded breeds, which appear to react less to their environments and companions.

Things to look for:

∩ introversion;

∩ lack of enthusiasm;

∩ lack of response to their surroundings and other horses.

Rescue™ Remedy (39)

Rescue™ Remedy is the best-known trade name for a combination of five remedies ready-mixed for emergency use. The remedies in it are:

- Star of Bethlehem (shock);
- Clematis (faintness, lack of focus);
- Rock Rose (terror and panic);
- Cherry Plum (loss of self-control);
- Impatiens (agitation and irritability).

Rescue™ Remedy can be thought of as a single remedy with its own indications, which is why it is sometimes referred to as the 39th remedy. It can help whenever a horse under pressure needs some help to stay calm and in control.

Riders and owners often give Rescue™ Remedy to horses because it is an obvious way of helping them keep calm in difficult situations. This does not mean it is a panacea for all ills. Once the immediate stress has been dealt with, the long-term solution lies in mixing an individual combination of remedies for your particular, individual horse. There is no danger involved in using Rescue™ Remedy over a long period of time, but it is unlikely to cure deep-seated imbalances – for that you need to turn to the system of 38 remedies.

Times to use Rescue™ Remedy include:

- before and during any stressful event;
- emergencies that leave the horse dazed, disorientated, frightened, upset, etc.;
- any first-aid situation in which there is no time to make a balanced assessment.

Rescue™ Cream

Rescue™ Cream is a soft, non-greasy, lanolin-free cream. It contains Rescue™ Remedy and Crab Apple, which is chosen for its cleansing qualities. It is usually applied to physical problems such as skin disorders, rashes, minor cuts, bruises and so on.

The cream might appear to be an exception to the rule that says that the remedies treat emotional states. But in fact it is simply a convenient way of applying Rescue™ Remedy and Crab Apple externally, in much the same way as a practitioner might give a mix of remedies selected for an emotional state and apply the same remedies in a compress to any external manifestation of the underlying emotional disorder. The kind of problems Rescue™ Cream treats are usually accompanied by some form of emotional stress or crisis (which explains why Rescue™ Remedy is in the cream), or by a feeling of contamination and dislike of one's own appearance (which accounts for the presence of Crab Apple). Just as Rescue™ Remedy would be useful for someone who has fallen downstairs, so the cream can be used to treat the external manifestation of the crisis.

Rescue™ Cream is available in two sizes. For humans the most common size is a 30-g tube, but if you want to use it on your horses you would be better off with the 400-g tub, which you can order direct from the makers (see the addresses section on page 201). Just smear the cream onto the affected area to more than cover it, and repeat as often as required. You shouldn't use the cream or anything else on open or deep wounds without consulting the vet first, and remember in all cases of physical injury or disease that Rescue™ Cream can't replace professional advice.

Selecting for horses

We carry about with us a filter constructed by our upbringing and our imbibed culture. It influences the way we see the world and makes it difficult for us to look at life through the eyes of someone from a different culture. Business people from one country making deals with business people from other countries often go on courses to help them communicate. Even a shared language and history is no guarantee of a shared worldview, which is why English people and Americans so often find each other puzzling. Does an investment banker fully understand the worldview of a punk, that of a nun, a refugee or a porn star? If cultural barriers within our species are so high, we would expect an even greater barrier between species.

This is indeed what we find. Horses and humans are divided by body shape and by their roles in life. The main problem we will face when using the remedies on horses is knowing how they see the world. The temptation is to assume that they *are* 'just like us' and select on that basis. We can have some limited success with this approach, because in some ways horses are 'just like us'. Certainly, as we will see in a moment, both species share some basic abilities. But in many crucial ways horses are very much unlike people, just as each individual horse is unlike the rest of the herd. If we fail to understand the differences we will inevitably misunderstand their needs, and we will approach them wrongly and select the wrong remedies. In this section we will sketch in the fundamental considerations that we need to have in mind when we look at horse behaviour in general, and at the behaviour of any one individual horse in particular. These basic concepts will be built and elaborated on in Part Two.

Predators and prey

According to current thinking different parts of the mammalian brain correspond to different functions. Researchers have drawn up maps showing which areas deal with sensory data, which with pain, and so on. Comparing the brains of different animals, it turns out that all mammals, from rabbits to horses to people, have very similar brains. We share the mechanisms that enable most kinds of intelligence, including emotional intelligence and the ability to learn. It is only reasonable to assume, unless proved otherwise, that we also share the intelligences themselves. In other words, horses are no different from 'higher' mammals like us in that they can learn and feel emotions. Indeed, the same proportion of the total brain mass is devoted to emotions in both humans and horses. This supports our assumption that horses are capable of the same number and intensity of emotions as we are.

As we have seen, however, 'just like us' overstates the case. Staying with the brain, we find a much smaller proportion of the equine brain is devoted to rational thought. This suggests horses do not analyse and brood over their feelings to the extent that we do and so tend not to carry as much emotional baggage, and would explain why horses often react well to well-chosen remedies. The practitioner doesn't usually need to dig down through layers of unresolved angst and rationalisation to find the central issue. Instead, the main difficulty lies in making that first selection. And again we come back to the same question: how exactly do we select remedies for horses?

A useful start is to think about horses in general and the way they live and interact. All horses share a fundamental approach to life, just as all people are human and look at life in a human way. If you can empathise with your horse's view of the world you can get a feel for the kind of emotions that he might feel in whatever situation he finds himself.

The first thing to keep in mind at all times is that humans are predators, but horses are prey animals. This explains many of the differences in the horse's way of seeing events in the world. If we want to understand our horses we need to make a real and sustained effort to think like a prey animal. And this means understanding what motivates them.

When something threatening happens to any prey animal, he

has four possible responses: run away, freeze, fiddle about (see page 101) or fight. But running away will always be his first choice. So the first motivation for a horse is his need to be able to escape from danger. Speed of flight is his main protection against being eaten. He needs somewhere to run to and as good a view as possible of the horizon so he can see anything trying to sneak up on him and get a good head start. A cave or building is not a naturally safe hide-out, as it is for us and other predators, but a potential trap.

The second motivation is social, and relates to the safety found in a herd. Horses look for the freedom to be part of a society that includes a pair-bond and other secondary relationships. With the first two motivations in mind, we begin to see why so many horses have a problem with stables. How can they be comfortable if they can't see all around them so as to check there are no tigers sneaking up, and if they have to stay on guard 24 hours a day because there is nobody else to take a turn at keeping lookout? Social life is also part of the third motivation: the need to play. Playing strengthens social bonds and keeps the horse alert. Fourth is the freedom to eat...and eat...and eat – for like all large herbivores horses have to spend a very large amount of time eating in order to get the nutrients and energy they need. Even if we are feeding them concentrated food that is supposed to meet their nutritional needs, horses still feel the drive to eat all the time. Artificial diets tend to ignore the behavioural side of feeding.

Humans in general seem to find it much easier to understand and empathise with other meat eaters. One only has to look at the number of cats and dogs kept as pets, compared with rabbits and other herbivores, to see this preference at work. We are so accustomed to being predators that it takes a real effort to empathise with horses. But it can be done. Two outstanding examples of people who have achieved wonders in this area are the famous horse trainer, Monty Roberts, and ex-rodeo champion Pat Parelli.

In his autobiography *The Man Who Listens to Horses*, Monty Roberts tells how he learned to communicate using a visual horse language while working for his father in California in the 1940s. He called this language 'Equus'. Roberts uses Equus to reassure and work with unbroken horses. Instead of punishing them into submission he uses his body posture and the making and breaking of eye contact to 'argue' them into a position of trust.

Heather Simpson is the founder of a system called Positive Horse Magic. This relies on positive reinforcement and a knowledge of equine behaviour to set up natural communication systems between horse and rider. A rider who uses this system does not have to use bits and whips to control her mount. Instead she aims to build up a partnership with the horse, so that rider and horse do things together because they both want to do the same thing.

The success of these methods demonstrates that horses and humans do indeed share ideas about relationships, trust and loyalty. When we look closely at the way horses feel about each other, about their lives, and about us, we can see our own personality types and emotional patterns mirrored in theirs, despite the fundamental distances between predators and prey. The triggers for emotions might be different – horses and humans get upset over different things – and we might express our upset in different ways. But the actual upsets – fear, jealousy, impatience, intolerance – are as closely related as lung and brain function and the purpose of muscles.

Understanding Equus

It's a good idea to learn some basic Equus if you want to select remedies for your horse. This will help you read your horse's feelings more accurately, and the more accurate you are the better your selection will be.

Let's start with sound, which is the communication system we humans identify with most readily. We can identify a number of specific sounds made by horses, including nickering, neighing, blowing and snorting, squealing, and roaring or screaming. None of these sounds have fixed meanings because a lot depends on the context in which they are used, but we can draw some general conclusions.

The nicker is basically a 'hello' or 'come here' sound. There are three subdivisions: the low guttural sound used to welcome friends and friendly humans; the longer and more broken sound a stallion makes to a desirable mare; and the soft call that mares use to get their foals to follow them. Neighing or whinnying is the classic horse noise – it starts with a squeal and ends with a nicker, with a grunt added at the end by stallions. People sometimes interpret this sound as a sign of fear, but it is more accurate to say it is a call used to establish contact with the herd. A rough translation might be, 'Hey, it's me!' Every horse has a slightly different neigh. Horses can tell who is calling and show more interest when the caller is their own foal or pair-bond or another herd member.

Squealing is a protest against something. You will sometimes hear it when a horse is suffering aggression or unwanted attention. A squeal warns the other horse that retaliation will follow if he doesn't stop. Mares often squeal during courtship, so the reading here could be that the mare is flirting, and pretending to be offended as a kind of come-on.

The sound of air blown out through the nostrils is a fairly neutral sign of interest or general well-being. When it turns into a snort and you can hear the nostrils vibrating this means that the horse is in two minds about something, displaying a mix of interest and anxiety, and possibly getting ready to run away. As for the roar and the higher-pitched scream, they are basically the same sound, and signal a very intense emotion such as fear or anger. Stallions may use roaring as a macho way of saying hello.

While it may be harder for us to understand and use, the most flexible part of Equus is not sound but body language. Here again context is all-important. Most of the time ear position simply indicates what a horse is listening to, or from what direction a sound has come, and a swishing tail may only mean that the midges are biting. But in other contexts, ears, tails, legs, and the position and direction of the body all have something to say to the careful observer. We can be fairly sure of our interpretation when these movements occur without an obvious neutral explanation, or when several types of body language are signalling the same thing.

Ears act like semaphores. Their position perched at the top of the head makes them especially important communicators because they can be seen from a distance. They let other horses in the herd know what their owner is interested in as well as signalling mood and intention. The 'at rest' position is to hold them upright, pointing forward and a little out to either side. This gives the best possible coverage of the area around the horse, so that he can hear any potential danger. A horse carrying his ears like this is not especially concerned about anything in the environment. But as soon as something happens – an unexpected noise, or a movement – the horse pricks and turns the nearest ear, or both ears, to point

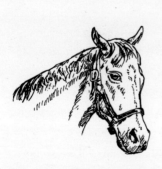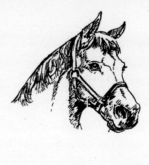

towards it. Eyes tend to follow ears, and the head and then the body soon follow if there seems an especial reason to be concerned. The concern shown by pricked ears isn't always fear due to a potential threat, however. You will also see pricked ears in animals who are interested in something pleasant such as a groom bringing food or the arrival of a friend. Real stress is shown by extremely pricked ears beginning to flick about.

The ears of tired, bored or depressed horses may droop down and stick out on each side of the head like birds' wings, the back of each ear at the top and the opening facing the ground. Or they may droop completely so that they hang down by the face. This position is also used to indicate submission and a lack of threat to dominant horses and riders. If your horse lets his ears droop when you are riding but turns them towards you this might suggest his feelings for you are a mix of submission (drooping) and fear (facing). The same ear position is sometimes seen in mares in season approaching feared and desired stallions. Drooping ears may also indicate that the horse feels some physical pain, so it's worth getting the advice of a vet if you notice your horse holding his ears like this over any length of time.

Don't confuse the sideways flop of the submissive horse with the flattened-back ears of aggression. When your horse pins his ears backwards along his neck so as to make them all but disappear this means he is threatening to attack. Pinned back they are less likely to be injured in battle. Before you reach for Vine and Holly, however, remember that the most common reason for aggression in a prey animal is fear compounded by an inability to escape. (See page 119 for more on aggression.)

With such large mobile ears, it is no surprise that horses hear better than humans. And this explains why they have less resistance to noise pollution than we do.

Turning to tails, we have mentioned that a lot of the time horses use them to keep flies and other irritations at bay. They are also a useful ballast and counterweight while moving around. But as communicators they are used even more than ears. In stationary horses a high tail indicates alertness and readiness to act, a droopy tail tiredness, pain, fear and submission. A horse out to enjoy himself may loop his tail right over his back, inviting others to join in. Aggressive horses may stick their tails straight out behind them to make themselves look bigger and more dangerous. And irritated, frustrated, unsettled horses may swish their tails in every direction, the flicks getting stronger and more decided as irritation turns into anger.

Tail swishing as a mood signal may be based on the action of swishing flies away. Horses use it as a kind of metaphor: 'I'm so upset it's like being bitten by midges.' The same seems to be true of some head movements. Horses move their heads away from danger and things they don't like, and by extension tossing or shaking the head indicate irritability in certain situations, as does head jerking, where the head moves up and back. But again there are many nuances. If the animal is being approached from behind, then tossing the head up and to the side can be a sign of submission. Aggressive horses thrust their heads forward as if to bite. A nudge is a similar forward movement but with a closed mouth – it too is assertive, but gentler, and is used to get attention. An upright head and neck shows alertness, and the head lowers into relaxation and slumps into depression and tiredness. Remember, though, that horses' eyes work differently from ours. Many head movements are to do with the way they focus on things, and this applies in particular to continuously bobbing the head down and up again. Other repetitive head movements may occur in depressed or psychologically damaged individuals – weaving the head from side to side, for example, can be the horse's equivalent of the continual rocking of a traumatised child (see page 106).

Body posture and direction are often used to display dominance. Moving into the path of another horse forces the victim to push on and risk a confrontation or move aside and accept second place. Horses will also jostle others with their shoulders to stress their dominance. Very dominant horses may reinforce their position by body-checking other horses.

In some animals turning the back towards an aggressor is a way of signalling submission. Horses are different because they generally defend with their rear hooves. Presenting the rump lines up a potential defensive kick and sends the message, 'Leave me alone – or else.' Lifting a back leg underlines the threat. In contrast, horses usually make aggressive attacks with their *front* hooves, sometimes rearing up to get close to their opponent. So a lifted front leg may indicate an aggressive threat – 'Just you watch it!' – although again this is not certain, as the same movement often indicates doubt and uncertainty. Stamping the back or front legs is more definite. Just as when we stamp our feet, this translates into a protest: 'Stop it!' or 'I don't want to!' And while horses often paw the ground to test the surface, this can also be a sign of frustration or depression, especially in an animal who wants to move on but can't for some reason.

Mouth, nostrils and eyes all show mood, just as they do in humans. Tense, anxious animals, or those in pain, have tense mouths. Relaxed or tired horses hold their mouths loosely. The lower lip actually droops down in very sleepy horses. Your horse may also relax his mouth to display submission to a more dominant horse. Chewing motions can show meekness or contentment, but if they are very fast they may indicate anxiety. Tense open jaws are a threat to bite. Flared nostrils show interest and readiness for action, although Arab horses are just built this way, which is why they look especially lively even when they are tired. Angry horses turn their eyes to the back, showing the white, and you will also see more white if the horse is frightened. Dominant horses stare directly at rivals so as to intimidate them.

As you can see, Equus is as complicated as any other language. Speaking it like a native takes years of dedication. But with practice and patience you can learn the basic vocabulary and gain genuine insight into the social life and mood of your horse.

Breed, sex and personality

For thousands of years humans have selected which animals will be allowed to breed. We know that by picking the parents we will be able to enhance features like intelligence, calmness, strength and body shape in their young. Every animal comes as a package, however, with a set of characteristics, some of which are desirable and some not so desirable. When we enhance the desirable features we also inadvertently enhance the undesirable ones.

We can see the results of our intervention most clearly in that most varietal of animals, the dog. Each breed has been created for a particular purpose. Often the purpose involves physical shape and prowess. But along the way different breeds have also acquired definite breed personalities, made up of a mix of positive and negative character traits that their selected ancestors happened to display. Some traits have been bred for deliberately. Others have emerged inadvertently.

Over centuries breeders have selected horses in exactly the same way. They have tried to improve their ability to pull, or carry, or jump, or race. Because of this similarity of approach, we might expect to be able to discover a genetic tendency towards this or that personality in each of the equine breeds, as we could with dogs. And we can, to an extent, although there are two important reservations.

The first is that breed personalities in horses are harder to define than they are in dogs, at least from our point of view. When Elwyn Hartley Edwards tries to assign definite characteristics to the breeds listed in *The Ultimate Horse Book,* he uses words like 'calm', 'tractable' and 'cooperative' over and over again. The observations lack explanatory force. The problem is the one we have already identified: we find it much easier to understand dogs because we are both predators. The nuances of personality in a prey animal are far more alien.

The second is that we need to be wary in any case about making hard and fast judgements. Sorting horses into personality types on the basis of physique and ancestry is like dividing humanity according to ethnic type: tall, rational, cool-headed Scandinavians on the one hand; slighter, hot-blooded, vivacious Latins on the other. It is a wide generalisation that we need to take with a very large pinch of salt.

That said, the broadest distinctions turn out to be the most helpful out in the field. The first and most obvious is between the athletic breeds such as Arabs and thoroughbreds, and bigger heavier types like Shire horses and Friesians. The former are known as 'hot-blooded' horses, come from the south, and tend to be more excitable and irritable and unpredictable. The latter are 'cold-blooded', come from the north, and tend to be stolid and slow to rouse. (The Latin/Scandinavian opposition raises its head again.) 'Warm-bloods', like the stocky horses known as cobs, are a mix of hot and cold. Their build lies somewhere between the hot- and cold-blood.

A cob is not, properly speaking, a breed at all but a description of a particular body shape. Some authorities nevertheless characterise horses of this shape as steady, slow to panic and willing, with a tendency to be dull and greedy. Coat colour is sometimes associated with behaviour as well – you will find piebald horses described as especially intelligent, good-tempered and hard-working.

Ponies – small horses of under 14.2 hands in height – tend to be hardier and stronger than the average horse. They may be less nervy and in some ways more independent, prepared to refuse your orders if they conflict with equine common sense. Tiny animals who have the slender legs and slighter build of horses are often called 'miniature horses' to differentiate them from 'true' ponies.

The sex of the horse may be another pointer towards personality tendencies. Traditionally stallions are described as headstrong and difficult to handle. In most circles only the most experienced handlers ride them. There is some truth in this, and we go into the subject further in Part Two. Nevertheless, human traditions and social customs have coloured the view we have of stallions and have led us to endow them with some tendencies that they do not in fact possess. For example, it is common practice to keep stallions away from foals for fear that they might stamp on them and kill them. Yet in the wild stallions are very tolerant of playing foals, just like the vast majority of adult horses. The problem only arises in our stallions because we raise them in solitary confinement and deny them the chance to learn normal social behaviour.

It comes as a surprise to many people to learn that herds of wild horses are run and led by a dominant *female*. The alpha (or breeding) male acts as a protector of his herd when other males try to muscle in, and fusses about to keep the herd together, but the alpha mare decides when the herd will move and where to, and assumes responsibility for herd discipline. Mares are not shrinking violets, and some individuals are especially inclined to play up when in heat. Hence the view shared by many that male geldings are generally steadier than mares.

Breed, conformation and sex may suggest which types of personality and behaviour are more likely than others, but it is clear they will not let us predict behaviour and personality with any certainty when we look at an individual horse. All horses are capable of all kinds of horse behaviour, and any of the 38 remedies could apply to any horse, regardless of other considerations. So having thought about horses in general and having given some consideration to the breed and conformation and sex of your horse, we need to take a further step.

Type remedies

The further step takes us into the heart of remedy selection.

Start by thinking about the particular horse you want to help. What tells him apart from every other horse? How would you describe his natural temperament: is he aggressive, or highly strung, or sociable, or loving, or gentle? Think about how he tends to act when things go wrong: does he go very quiet and withdrawn, or does he protest? Is he assertive and extrovert, or introvert and put-upon?

The answers to these questions will guide you towards probable *type remedies* for your horse. A type remedy is a remedy that describes a horse's fundamental personality and by extension tells you how he will probably feel whenever he is out of balance, either through illness or because of life's slings and arrows.

To get you thinking about your horse, here is a list of the most commonly used horse type remedies.

- Mimulus – shy, timid, nervous types who quickly take fright;

- Impatiens – quick-thinking, impetuous types who are always in a hurry and get irritable if they are held up;

- Vine – boss horses who know what they want and use force of character to get it;

- Chicory – give a lot of love, but sulk if they don't get enough attention from their humans, foals and equine friends;

- Beech – intolerant of different approaches, new things, grooming, touching, etc.;

- Vervain – enthusiastic horses who throw themselves into their favourite pursuits without considering the cost;

- Centaury – born followers and helpers, they are easily dominated and abused;

- Heather – types who hate being ignored, yet ignore the needs of others;

- Scleranthus – eternal ditherers, going from one thing to another without making up their minds either way;

- Clematis – excessively dreamy, sleepy types who seem to need more than the average horse's five-minute naps;

- Wild Rose – easy-going drifters who don't often get enthusiastic about life or anything in it;

- Water Violet – horses who seem especially happy with their own company and avoid spending time with all but a couple of select individuals;

- Agrimony – sociable horses who enjoy playing and romping so much it is sometimes hard to tell when they are unhappy;

- Larch – horses who avoid challenges and don't try to cope with difficulties;

- Oak – strong, slow, dependable, deliberate horses who do not know when they are beaten;

- Crab Apple – fussy, obsessive horses.

As with all remedy descriptions, many of these stress the negative. We don't need to be so exact about positive characteristics because a horse who feels positive doesn't need a remedy. And each type does indeed have its positive, balanced aspect. A positive Vine is a wise and restrained leader, a positive Heather a great companion and sharer of sorrows, a positive Beech a tolerant, understanding friend and neighbour.

Mood remedies

Having thought about his personality, there is one final step. Ask yourself how your horse seems right now. Is he particularly sleepy, hyperactive, aggressive, frightened or lethargic? Does he seem to be afraid of something, or look as if he has had a shock, or have no energy, or want to be fussed over, or want to be left alone? Have you noticed anything in particular that seems to be associated with this behaviour? Has something in the field or stable changed? Is this the first time your horse has seen a vet or had his tail plaited? Does he always get overexcited or anxious when a particular person rides him or when you visit certain places, or at the sight of his food or tack or the horsebox?

Questions like these will guide you to the *mood remedies* your horse needs. A mood remedy is a remedy that matches the way your horse feels at the moment. So while an Impatiens-type horse will tend to get irritable whenever there is a delay, any horse can be in an Impatiens state given the right circumstances. One individual might need Impatiens at feeding time, while another will only need it on the way to a show, or while waiting to be turned out for the day.

All of the 38 remedies can be mood remedies.

Selection in a nutshell

To sum up, selecting remedies means using your powers of observation, plus your knowledge of horses in general and of your horse in particular, plus a good dose of gut feeling, intuition and common sense, in order to determine as far as you can your horse's current state of mind. Once you think you know how he feels and why he is acting the way he is, you just select the remedies that match.

Don't worry if this seems complicated, because you do not need to overanalyse. If in doubt, keep things simple and treat what you see. If your horse does not need one of the remedies you give him, then that remedy will have no effect. Even if you select all the wrong remedies at least you know that they are positive in their essence, and will never make things worse.

Giving remedies to horses

Basic dosage for horses is the same as for humans. Add four drops of Rescue™ Remedy and/or two drops of any of the 38 remedies into a 30ml. (1oz.) dropper bottle filled with water. Use mineral water for preference, as this keeps fresh for longer. You can mix from one to seven remedies together at a time. If you include Rescue™ Remedy in a mix it counts as one remedy – so you could mix Rescue™ Remedy with up to six others.

A single dose from a mixed dosage bottle is four drops, given by mouth. Use any way of getting the drops into the mouth that works, but be careful of using the glass dropper directly because it may break or be swallowed. Many people give remedies by

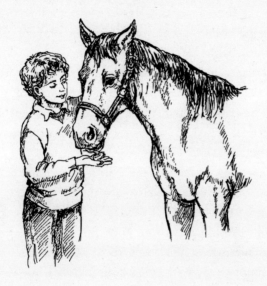

dropping them onto a quarter of apple or a piece of carrot sliced lengthways. Most horses are more than happy to accept this as a treat. Or you can drip the remedy mix around your horse's muzzle so that he licks it off.

You should give doses at regular intervals, and give at least four doses a day. You can give more frequent doses if you want, and doing so can be a good way of getting through a crisis.

Another approach is to add undiluted remedies to your horse's drinking water. The dosage for Rescue™ Remedy is about ten drops per bucket of fresh water. Your horse will then get a reasonable dose each time he drinks, even if he only takes a quick slurp. You can do the same with one or a combination of the 38 individual remedies as well – the dosage being five drops of each one. Just add further doses of the remedies each time you change the water.

If this is a problem – if your horse drinks from a stream, say, or you have an automatic water feeder – you can add the same quantities of remedies to his food instead. One way to do this is to mix the remedies with water in a mister – the kind used to freshen up plants – and spray hay nets or piles of hay or concentrate with this.

You can give undiluted remedies in an emergency, or when there is no water around. The effects are no stronger and it will cost you more money, but there is no danger involved in giving concentrated remedies. Some horses do not like the taste or smell of the brandy in the stock bottle.

The common idea behind these different methods of dosage is to make it convenient for you to give the remedies, and easy and stress-free for your horse to take them. You can use any method that you want as long as your horse gets at least the equivalent of a minimum dose: four drops from a dosage bottle, four times a day. Your horse will not overdose on remedies, nor will he build up tolerance or dependency. He needs to take enough remedy, but it does not matter if he takes more than he needs.

You and other humans

Caring owners also suffer when their horses are ill or unhappy, and may get so wrapped up in selecting and giving remedies that they forget to think about their own needs. Here are some obvious helpers for when you need support with your own feelings.

- Red Chestnut for anxiety about your horse's welfare;

- Star of Bethlehem for shock, either after an accident or when the vet has diagnosed a serious illness;

- Gentian for despondency, or Gorse if you feel very pessimistic;

- White Chestnut for constant worry;

- Agrimony if you try to put a brave face on things but feel upset underneath;

- Vervain for anger and frustration at the injustice of it all, or Willow if your anger is laced with self-pity;

- Impatiens if you feel agitated and impatient and want the problem to go away at once;

- Pine if you blame yourself for some act or omission that has caused the problem or made it worse.

Your horse will benefit if you take the time to help yourself with the remedies. You will be able to think more clearly and be more objective about selecting remedies for him. And he will feel better and calmer if you and his other carers are in balance, for just as an animal's distress can trigger distress in carers so the reverse is true. Distressed carers cause distress to their animals. Emotions like anxiety are infectious, and if you feel full of fear or tension your horse will empathise with your feelings and start to mirror your own state of mind. The old joke that people and their animals come to look like each other may not be true, but they certainly tend to share each other's neuroses. Indeed, you may be looking for remedies to help your horse when in fact your horse's emotional state is simply a manifestation of your own. Bearing in mind one of the most important principles of Dr Bach's work – treat the cause, not the effect – the remedies you want to give to your horse may be the remedies that you should be taking yourself.

This principle applies particularly to the problems experienced by novice riders. It's natural for us to feel anxious and unsure of ourselves when we first start riding. We sit in a tense position, pull on the reins for dear life so as to point the horse where we want to go, give contrary instructions with our aids, and sweat more than usual. Horses are very sensitive to vibration and to smell – that's how they identify members of their own herd – and react accordingly. If the rider is anxious and confused there must be something to be anxious and confused about. The horse gets agitated and starts looking for danger. This makes him more difficult to control. A vicious circle kicks in as the horse's skittish behaviour increases our fear, which in turn gets the horse even more upset.

The way to break the circle is to take some remedies ourselves before we get on the horse – such as Mimulus for our fear, or Larch for our lack of confidence. That way we will feel more relaxed and in control. Our confidence will inspire confidence in the horse. Even those of us who are very experienced riders might be surprised at what we could achieve with a little self-analysis and the use of a few well-chosen remedies.

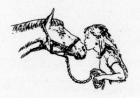

Part Two

Treating equine emotions

Two important reminders

In this part of the book we will look in much more detail at some of the situations horses find themselves in, and at the kind of responses they are likely to feel. Where we suggest remedies our aim is to point you towards remedies that you could usefully consider as a first step. Always remember, however, that your horse is an individual. He will not always react in exactly the same way as all other horses, and remedies that we have not mentioned may be central to his particular state of mind.

Go back to page 51 and the section headed 'Selecting for horses' if you are still unsure how to select remedies for your own individual horse.

Horses are often the victims of human thoughtlessness. Their first inclination when under stress is to move away. Nevertheless, they are bigger and stronger than humans, and often they have nowhere to move to. Any animal will attack if he feels that he has no choice.

We strongly advise you to give thought at all times to your own personal safety, and to be aware of the limits to your knowledge and skill. You should seek professional advice from qualified behaviourists and veterinary surgeons whenever necessary.

Emotion and behaviour

Horses and horses

As we saw earlier on in this book, horses are one of the many types of prey animals who choose to live in herds. Herd life has a number of advantages if you are a potential meal. First, herd members can look out for each other. A single horse has only one pair of eyes and one pair of ears and one set of nostrils with which to pick up the approach of a predator. A herd has many more chances of doing this successfully. Second, from the point of view of any one horse, it's quite likely that an attacking predator will get one of the others. If a horse were grazing by himself when a predator happened by he would be the only target. Herd life also provides more opportunities to play and practise life skills. And it implies a greater range of choice when it comes to reproducing, and a safer and more educational environment for bringing up offspring.

In the wild, herds of horses roam over massive ranges. This means that they don't usually need to compete for resources. If two herds happen to be in the same space at the same time they will normally avoid each other and move on. When food or water are scarce or in one place, however, herds may start to become more territorial and to compete with each other. Rival stallions may clash to settle which herd will claim living space. Similar kinds of space pressures can apply in stables and paddocks as well. While some horses accept newcomers and make friends, others may resent new arrivals and attack so as not to have to share limited resources.

Space and distance are big issues for horses. On the one hand they need to ensure that they can flee before a predator or another more aggressive horse gets too close. On the other hand they do not want to have to run every time something moves on the horizon. Doing so would use up valuable energy and eat into time that would be better used for grazing and social interaction. They need a complex sense of the space around them in order to balance these competing needs and respond appropriately to different levels of threat.

Behaviourists break up the horse's sense of space into four zones of various size. The first and smallest is *personal space*, which can be defined as the space that a horse uses when he stands, turns, lies down or stretches. *Pair-bond space*, as its name suggests, is the space occupied by a horse and his closest equine companion. It is also the distance that the pair keeps between itself and other horses. The distance between an *individual* horse and others who are not part of a pair bond is slightly different, and is referred to as *social space*. Finally the largest zone is *security space*, or *critical flight space*. This is defined by the area into which a potential aggressor has to move before the horse will run away.

Horses are careful about moving into each other's spaces. You will see one horse approach another at an angle. He may stop for a time, or even move backwards, before moving forwards again. All this gives the horse being approached a chance to evaluate the approaching horse and know that he is not a threat. When they do get close to each other they will often seal the greeting by blowing into each others' nostrils to exchange scent, which is analysed in hollow chambers called vomeronasal organs.

As well as being a way of cementing a friendship, swapping breath can also be an exchange of calling cards between potential rivals, helping them to decide which is likely to be dominant. Fights may break out if they are well matched, but battles are more thunder than blood. Loud roars are followed up by kicks, but these behaviours are designed to defuse aggression and horses rarely do real damage to each other. More submissive horses will mouth and snap their teeth to demonstrate that they are not trying to move up the pecking order.

Horses don't have a formal dominance hierarchy like that of dogs. Instead, context is very important in defining which animal will be dominant over another at a particular time. This is because dominance is not purely about deciding who is boss. It is also about how much a particular horse cares about a particular thing. For example one horse may be dominant over another when hay is distributed because he places particular value over feeding first and so asserts himself at that point. But if he isn't especially thirsty, he will happily wait his turn at the water bucket, allowing a more thirsty horse to go first even if he is usually dominant over that animal.

A horse's overall position in the herd is determined largely by the number of times he is able to demonstrate his dominance over others. But at the higher levels of dominance – such as alpha mare – dominant animals actually have less need to prove themselves. They know their own strength and authority, and show their confidence by putting more stress on the need to keep the herd stable and united. In effect, true leadership in the equine world is not so very different from leadership in the human world. It is tolerant and forgiving, and slow to anger. Stronger and more dominant horses in a herd often look after the interests of smaller, younger and weaker animals by driving away boisterous individuals who come too close. Only less confident animals have to assert themselves all the time.

A crucial contextual (and complicating) factor in herd dominance relationships is the phenomenon of pair-bonding, in

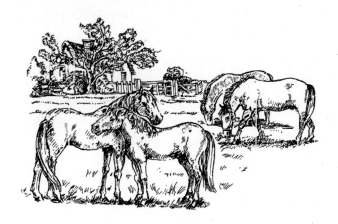

which a horse will form a strong life-long bond with one particular friend within the herd. Pair-bonds look out for each other, so both members of the pair feel safer and can take it in turns to rest and relax. They feed together. They play together, nipping and chasing and pushing against each other. They groom each other more than they groom other members of the herd, and they tend to stick together as they move around the field. Two pair-bonded horses may occupy very different positions in the herd, but the status of the subordinate will be raised when he acts in concert with his more dominant companion.

In the absence of other equines, horses may pair-bond with other species, such as goats and sheep, or even natural enemies like dogs, cats or humans. But horses that are kept in stables and are turned out by themselves do not have the opportunity to pair-bond with anyone. This can lead to emotional problems including anxiety, aggression and depression. Even having an odd number of horses in a herd can cause problems, because the odd-horse-out will not be able to pair-bond.

The complexity of herd relationships means that it is important not to disrupt a settled herd unnecessarily. If your horse establishes a place in the local herd try to keep the herd together by synchronising turn-out times and stabling with other owners.

Here are some suggestions to get you thinking about possible remedy solutions for when inter-horse relationships break down:

- ∩ Try Beech for horses who cannot tolerate the presence of others, and chase them away or kick out to show their displeasure.

- ∩ Choose Vine for very dominant horses who bully others.

- ∩ Select Centaury for submissive horses who tend not to fight back or resist.

- Chicory is for affectionate horses who like to keep their particular friend to themselves.

- Give Holly to horses who show real spite towards others, or get jealous if another horse steals affection from one of their equine or human companions.

- Give Heather to horses who seem desperate for any company and follow others around even when rebuffed.

- Use Mimulus for shy, timid horses who avoid the company of louder or more extrovert animals.

- Give Larch to horses who seem to lack basic confidence.

- Walnut is to help adjust to any changes in the horse's relationships.

Stallions

Successful stallions want to protect their harem and its living space and keep it to themselves, but this doesn't mean that they are 'top dogs' in charge of everything, or that they are 'ruthless' or 'nasty'. As we have seen, mares take on the day-to-day running of the herd, and that includes herd discipline. The stallion follows along behind, only intervening when the herd risks scattering or when a challenger poses a threat to his position. Nevertheless only expert riders and trainers work with ungelded male horses. This is because, as horse owners, we find a lot of the things male horses do inconvenient and troublesome.

First of all, normal behaviour in male horses includes fighting other males. This starts when they are colts. Play-fighting is fun and a chance to let off steam, but it is also serious practice for when the grown-up stallion will need these skills in order to see off rivals. Normal play-fighting includes rearing up and biting, both of which understandably cause concern to horse owners and yard managers.

If rivalry with other males is one problem, the stallion's relationship with females is another. Stallions are not always gentle

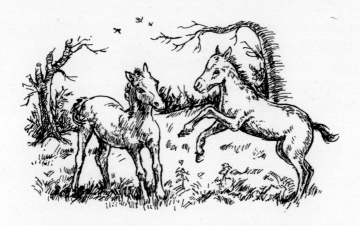

with their harem, and will threaten aggression and even bite in order to keep them in the group. Further handling problems arise because males are always looking to add to their collection of females – a fact of life which sometimes involves harassed owners in diplomatic incidents with the owners of mares.

A third major male characteristic has only recently come to light. We know that the male hormone testosterone controls the sex drive of horses and also causes their aggressive behaviour. It now seems that this same hormone inclines stallions to show more abstract qualities like determination and persistence. So when we feel intimidated by a stallion it is not just because they tend to be stronger and more powerful. We are also aware that the stallion has definite goals in mind and that these goals may not be ours. And he won't give up easily.

Stallions tend to be more alert than mares, so they notice what you are doing more quickly. They also tend to be bolder and to take more risks. This makes them more inclined to confront you if they think it is in their interest to do so. This is why situations that are easy to manage if your horse is a mare or a gelding can be highly charged and risky if your horse is an entire stallion. Imagine leading a gelding away from his herd – most of the time it is a simple and straightforward task. Now imagine leading a stallion in the same situation. To the stallion the herd may be *his* in a far stronger way. You are not just leading one horse away from a lot of others – you are leading a sheikh away from his harem. For all he knows as soon as he is away some other horse will come along and hijack them. He does not want to go, and he may decide that it is worth taking the risk of challenging you in order to achieve his goal.

Unless you are especially experienced at working with all types of horses, you are almost bound to use strict management routines on a stallion even if it is only to keep yourself safe from possible attack. Any livery yard owner is sure to insist on it, because otherwise the stallion's behaviour will draw complaints from his other customers.

When they are living natural lives in the wild, male horses always live in herds. If they are strong and successful they form their own herds of mares. If they are less successful they will live in a group with other bachelors. In either case they will enjoy the benefits of living with others – social contact, protection from danger, and play. But in yards they often end up living in solitary confinement until the end of their days. This is unnatural and dangerous to their mental and emotional health. And the health risks don't stop there. Stallions feel an immense drive to seek out other horses, and because they are natural risk-takers they may try to escape from their secure accommodation and end up with severe injuries as a result.

For all these reasons the stock advice to anybody owning a colt is to have him gelded. Gelding softens male behaviour, so much so that many owners consider geldings to be even easier and more tractable than mares. The horse will have a better life under human care because the human will feel able to work with him in a less constrictive environment.

Indeed, the only good reason not to *geld* a colt is if you intend to breed horses. And even then there are reasons for thinking twice. Animal shelters kill dogs and cats every day of the week because there are no homes for them. Increasingly this is happening to horses too. Equine sanctuaries and rescue centres are having to take in more and more horses whose owners no longer want them. Because horses are not running wild in city streets the problem is far less discussed. But it is still pressing, and if we really are horse-lovers we need to look hard at any plans that might add to the problem.

Learning

Horses are intelligent because they act in ways that help meet their needs. Because their needs are different from ours, their intelligence does not necessarily make it easier for us to get what we want from them. We are right to assume that horses who do not automatically submit to our every unreasonable command might be more intelligent than their less spirited brothers. When dealing with intelligent horses we need to use our own intelligence if we want to meet them on equal terms. We need to find ways to communicate with them that encourage them to understand us and want the same things we want.

All behaviour can be divided into two types: instinctive and learned. Instinctive behaviour includes mating, playing and running – things all horses are born knowing how to do. Learned behaviour is based on the horse's experiences in life. It is because horses in general are so good at learning that we and they have formed such a long-lasting and flexible partnership; but just as with people, every individual horse learns in different ways and has different learning abilities. Five main factors influence learning aptitude, and we need to bear all of them in mind when deciding on the best approach to teaching something to our particular horse.

1. **Breed** – some breeds of horse are naturally more intelligent and aware than others. Hardy ponies tend to be calmer and less reactive than hot-blooded animals like thoroughbreds and Arabs. We would expect the latter to notice things faster but also to be less forgiving of bad practice on our part.

2. **Personality** – as with schoolchildren, some horses are better students than others.

3. **Past experiences** – we never start with a blank slate when we start training our horse, because he has already learned from his past experiences and will apply his knowledge to new situations. If he has had a bad experience with the bit it will be harder to get him used to it, and if he has been mistreated in general it will be harder (but not impossible) to teach him anything.

4. **Health** – the healthier the horse, the more curiosity he has and the more he is able to learn.

5. **Sexual state** – a mare in season and any nearby stallions are less likely to be interested in the rest of the environment.

We might add a sixth point, age, except that this is less important than you might think. Horses are built to learn every day, because in the wild they need to learn in order to survive. A horse who escapes a danger today by running away is more likely to survive tomorrow if he has learned not to put himself in that situation in the first place. Thanks to their commitment to life-long learning we can always teach new tricks to an old horse, although it may take a little more time and patience.

Perhaps the simplest form of learning is *habituation*. This means getting used to things – or, more exactly, learning to take no notice of things that don't make any real difference to us. Traffic whizzing by inches away from a crowded pavement is dangerous. Yet people who live in cities become habituated to the noise and rush and may actually find the silence of the countryside more disturbing. In the same way, it is natural for a horse to be frightened of a passing tractor because it is large and strange and may be dangerous. But if he lives on a farm and sees and hears tractors every day, sometimes in the distance and sometimes nearby, and slowly gets used to the smell and noise of them, he forms the view that tractors are neutral and can be ignored safely. He has become habituated to tractors.

Like all prey animals, horses need to use habituation in order to survive at all. This is how they learn that falling leaves, waving branches, and the noise of the wind are not dangerous. If they weren't able to learn this they would never be able to feed or sleep. Every movement and sound would have them running away just in case it was a tiger.

We can take advantage in several ways of our horses' natural tendency to habituate to things. We can help them get used to the various flight triggers that litter our artificial environments – whips, saddles, flapping flags and plastic bags, banging gates, and so on. We can help them overcome natural fears, such as their instinctive fear of snakes. From an evolutionary point of view, a fear of snakes is good news because it means the horse is less likely to get bitten. But from our point of view it can be undesirable if it leads the horse to panic every time he passes a garden hose. We can also habituate them to inherently frightening situations, such as hacking in traffic and having feet shod, although the latter can be especially tricky. A flight animal like a horse is sure to feel uncomfortable and anxious if he feels that he can't use his legs properly. This is why many techniques for loading horses onto trailers require a careful programme of habituation if they are to be successful. They rely on you being able to get a rope around the horse's legs without him getting unduly upset.

There are a couple of general rules that apply to habituation. The first is that the longer it takes to habituate a horse to something, the longer he will stay habituated. Rapid habituation may seem more decisive, but it invariably leads to relapses later on. The second is that the horse is habituated to the event or thing, and at the same time to the whole context in which it is set. What this means in practical terms is that you might successfully habituate your horse to your horse box at his home yard, and get to the competition and unload him and think you have solved the problem. But then at the end of the day he won't get back into the box. He sees the different surroundings as part of a wholly new situation in which it may no longer be safe to get into the box. To be truly 'cured' you have to habituate him to getting into and out of the box in enough different settings that it is the box, and not the yard, that he is used to.

Like any other learning process, habituation can be blocked if the horse has had a bad experience in the past. This is especially serious if the bad experience has *sensitised* the horse. Sensitisation is the opposite of habituation. A horse sensitised to a horse box is so frightened of it that he stops thinking completely. He freezes or panics, and is simply incapable of learning at all.

A second form of learning is called *conditioning*. We could think of conditioning as the process of creating associations in the horse's mind – except that this suggests that we always condition horses deliberately, and that is far from true. You might be in the habit of singing arias from *Carmen* when you arrive at 4.30 to give a daily treat to your horse. He will soon associate the time of day and your attempts at Bizet with the food. In other words, you will have conditioned him to expect food when he hears Bizet, in the same way that Pavlov conditioned his dogs to salivate at the ringing of a bell.

Unintentional conditioning can be the source of many problems. Perhaps an ill-fitting saddle or tight reins and a nervous rider have caused the horse pain during a competition. Next time he enters the competition ring he associates this action with the pain and begins to protest. Or maybe something has scared him while he is out on a hack. In his mind, the scare is associated with the feel of the bit in his mouth. His fear that the scare will happen again may be displaced into head-shaking or some other 'vice' next time you try to give him the bit.

If you suspect that your horse has been conditioned into misbehaving, your first step should be to have the vet check that there isn't another explanation. If all is well physically, start by identifying the cues that trigger the fear. Then you need to get the horse used to those triggers by dissociating them from the pain or the memory of the scare. This is called counter-conditioning. In the case of the head-shaking horse, for example, you might leave the bit hanging around and let him play with it, or rub it over his body. If your riding hat or clothes are the trigger, wear them when you are grooming or feeding him but have no intention of riding. If a particular stretch of bridleway is the trigger, try leading him down it instead of riding, or hacking along it at a different time of day. In all these cases, the aim is to break the link between the trigger (jingling bit, riding hat, etc.) and the response (fear that the scare will recur) by showing him that the trigger does not lead inevitably to any particular event. This takes patience, so don't be tempted to push him on too fast. The slower you go, the better the results will be in the end.

Habituation and counter-conditioning are largely passive approaches in which the horse is put into contact with something that could be dangerous and finds that nothing happens. After a time, he stops noticing it. A more active form of teaching is when we deliberately *reinforce* behaviours. There are two ways of reinforcing behaviour – *negative reinforcement* and *positive reinforcement*.

Negative reinforcement happens when an unpleasant result

accompanies a behaviour, but stops as soon as the the behaviour stops. A horse nibbles at an electric fence and receives a shock; when he stops nibbling the shock stops. He has been taught by negative reinforcement not to touch wires. A colt who tries to mount a mare gets a kick for his pains but she stops kicking when he moves away – he has been taught by negative reinforcement not to mount her again. A horse who doesn't want to move forward gets a pull from a lead rope but the pressure stops when he moves – he has been taught by negative reinforcement to move forward when asked. In each case, the horse doesn't like what is happening so he tries different things (not touching the fence, moving away from the mare, moving forward) until he finds one that makes it stop. Because he tries different things, negative reinforcement is also called trial-and-error learning.

Used judiciously, negative reinforcement is an effective way of teaching a horse to do what we want. But it is essential to remove the unpleasant consequence as soon as the unwanted behaviour stops. If we don't do this, the horse has no way of knowing when he has done the right thing. Imagine a horse being led across the yard. He moves forward, but the pressure from the halter doesn't stop. Because his first try didn't work, he tries something else – perhaps he shakes his head or tries to go sideways. The pressure is still there. Eventually, if nothing works, he just gives up and stops trying at all. The person tugging on the lead rope says that the horse is dull and unresponsive. She practically has to tow him when she wants to lead him. But it would be truer to say that she has taught him to be helpless and to ignore what she does, because nothing he does seems to influence her.

The same kind of self-defeating attempts at negative reinforcement are seen in riders who pull harder and harder on the bit to make a horse who is stopping stop faster, or who repeatedly kick to make a horse who is going fast go faster, or who keep flicking a lunge whip behind a moving horse to keep him moving. In each case, the horse is already doing what he is being asked to do. Repeating the negative reinforcer only causes confusion and stops the horse from learning.

The great risk of negative reinforcement is that it slides so easily into brute force and cruelty. In technical terms we can make a negative reinforcer so *salient* that the horse can't ignore it. This means that the negative reinforcer is so overriding that it is the main thing that the horse notices. He focuses on it and adjusts his behaviour accordingly, no matter what else is going on. We could imagine a horse bolting in panic. A straightforward pull on a straightforward bit may not be enough to overcome his need to run away. The simplest way for the rider to achieve saliency is to pull harder and use a harsher bit. Eventually the pain from the bit will be great enough to become more important to the horse than his fear. So he will stop. Understanding the real cause of the problem – in other words, why the horse is frightened in the first place – takes more time and skill. All a cruel bit takes is a few pounds and no imagination...

If negative reinforcement is the stick, positive reinforcement is the carrot. Positive reinforcement happens when a pleasant outcome follows a piece of behaviour. The positive outcome can be food, a friendly word, a pat, a toy – anything that the horse likes. As with negative reinforcement, he will only associate the reinforcement with the behaviour if the two follow immediately – in other words, within a second or two of each other.

It's easy to see how positive reinforcement can be used when a horse is spontaneously doing something that we want to encourage. But how do we use it when the horse is doing something that we don't want him to do? Often the answer is to ignore or interrupt the behaviour until it stops, then use positive reinforcement to reward the fact that it has stopped. So if your horse nips you while you are grooming him, you might push him away to interrupt the behaviour, then give him a stroke to reward him for not nipping.

Most of the time negative and positive reinforcement can be used together to good effect. For example, difficulties loading horses are fear-based. The horse is so frightened of getting into this metal box that his fear overrides most normal negative reinforcements. One answer would be to make his life so unutterably unpleasant that he prefers to get into the box in spite of his fear. Clearly this would be cruel and would not solve the real problem, which is his fear – as you will find out next time you try to load him. A better approach would be to reduce the horse's fear using positive reinforcement. Then at the point of loading you will only need to use mild negative reinforcement.

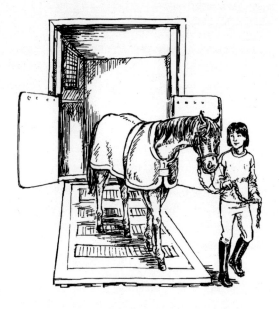

Because it is mild, it is more easily controlled, and you will be better able to reward the horse by removing it the instant he starts to move forward. You will know if you are being successful in your training if the horse does things more willingly the next time around.

All teachers have to learn when to stop a lesson. Ideally, any training session should end with a success and with praise for the horse. If something goes wrong, go back to the previous stage so as to finish with something that works. Then stop, take a rest, and if necessary rethink your strategy and objectives. You have to be honest with yourself as well, and know your own limits. Get help if a problem exceeds your competence. Get help if you feel at any time that a situation is beyond your control. And never take risks with your own safety – remember that however meek and mild he is, your horse is bigger and stronger than you and needs to be treated with respect.

- Chestnut Bud is associated with a failure to observe and learn from past mistakes. Consider it for your horse if he is slow to pick things up, and for yourself if you have trouble learning to teach.

- Impatiens can help you calm down and show more patience.

- Vine can help if you tend to use force to get your own way. Take it to help you appreciate better your horse's individual needs.

Abnormal behaviour

Many of the things we do to horses in the name of good management are abnormal in their eyes. Take saddling. Many experts introduce horses to the saddle as soon as they are strong enough to bear a rider's weight. This happens when the horse is about three or four years old, and usually coincides with stabling and of course with all the trappings of being ridden – bits, reins and bridles, and schooling and training. But for the horse this age is a milestone for a different reason. In the wild, a three-year-old is just finding his feet and beginning to feel confident. His interest in the world around increases, and he becomes intensely curious.

He wants to explore, to find things out. So he often reacts badly to his sudden confinement and lack of freedom. And, as if to make matters worse, as soon as he is in the stable and unable to run around we feed him on concentrated, energy-rich foods.

Saddling and stabling are only two of the ways in which our management routines and lack of understanding place the horse under stress. We control his social interaction with other horses, or deny him any contact with them at all. We invade his personal space without any invitation. We deprive him of 24-hour grazing, which is natural to him, and instead feed him two or three times a day, which is natural to us. We surround him with unusual sights and sounds and smells, yet do not give him the chance to investigate them for himself so as to find out what they are. We put him into strange situations such as competitions and schooling without habituating him to them first. And those of us who are not good riders inflict our poor seat, heavy hands and nervousness on him every time we get on his back.

Abnormal treatment like this will lead to abnormal behaviour if the horse loses his emotional balance and becomes agitated and clinically depressed. The sign that this is happening is the development of a number of stereotypical behaviours that we in our wisdom call *vices*. A vice – more usually called a *stable vice* because, for obvious reasons, it will especially afflict stabled horses – is any kind of irrational, meaningless behaviour that is repeated over and over. Common examples of vices in depressed horses are wind-sucking, crib-biting, fur-tugging, box-walking and weaving. In humans, the same conditions and mental states lead to rocking, head-banging, compulsive hand-washing, and so on. In both species, continued mental distress can impair the immune system, leading to infections, general poor health and weight loss. For more information, see the section on stereotypical behaviour on page 106.

Not all unwanted behaviour is abnormal in this way, of course. There is a much larger category of perfectly normal behaviours that just happen to be inconvenient for us. This includes the many types of response due to fear or lack of confidence. For example, a horse who has been startled by some perceived danger will bolt. This is natural. A horse being put into a situation that he thinks is dangerous will resist. This too is natural, as is napping, when a horse tries to return to the safety of his herd because he is not confident in his rider. In these cases, understanding, simple training techniques and well-chosen remedies can help reassure him that there is no need to worry.

∩ The main remedy for fear of a known thing is Mimulus. Aspen is for a more vague, more generalised fear that has no real locus.

∩ Larch can help horses that lack confidence.

∩ Crab Apple is good for obsessive behaviours including stereotypical behaviour.

∩ The long-term remedy for frustrated horses confined inside is 24-hour turn out. Vervain will help ease their frustration and overexuberance when they are first released.

∩ Walnut will help during any change of management.

Behavioural changes

Call the vet whenever a horse suddenly starts to behave differently or in unexpected ways. Many organic diseases cause a change in behaviour, and some of them are serious, such as tumours and hormonal problems. Remember too that many apparent behavioural problems are due to undiagnosed pain. Possible causes include ill-fitting or poorly designed tack, hoof and leg problems, ragged teeth cutting into the cheeks, and nervous riders pulling at the bit. A horse who suddenly seems shy or fractious could have suffered a hidden injury. If you check for pain and call out the vet as soon as your horse starts to behave differently, then you may be able to nip a physical problem in the bud before it becomes serious.

This doesn't mean that you can't use the remedies straight away, even before physical causes have been investigated, because they can only do good and will never make things worse. And once physical causes have been ruled out, you can give your full mind to the actual behaviour, and to the living conditions and emotional states that cause it. Any of the remedies could apply in different circumstances. Here are some suggestions to get you thinking.

- ∩ Give Scleranthus when there are sudden shifts of mood, from euphoria to melancholy and back again, or when the horse never seems to settle on an even keel.

- ∩ Try Aspen when your horse becomes fearful for no apparent reason, or suddenly starts to behave anxiously in normal, everyday situations. (Be aware that Mimulus is just as likely, since the cause may be clear to the horse even if it isn't clear to you.)

- ∩ Consider Crab Apple for horses who seem reluctant to eat or stale, and for horses who are distressed by skin or digestion problems.

- ∩ Try Mustard when your horse seems morose and depressed for no reason.

- ∩ Try Hornbeam if your normally lively horse seems to lack the energy to enjoy life. (Consider Wild Rose and Olive as well.)

- ∩ Choose Walnut if you can trace the change in behaviour to a change in the horse's life, such as a new management routine or a change of rider.

- ∩ Try Elm if your normally capable horse seems depressed following an increase in work or any other additional burden.

Mounting

Stallions mount mares when they are breeding. This much is obvious. But mounting also takes place at other times, and its meaning then is different. A mare who begins to mount other mares or develops other male characteristics may be suffering from an ovarian tumour and may require surgery. If you feel any concern you should want to call out the vet to check. But in most cases 'inappropriate' mounting is normal behaviour. For animals under three, it is usually role-playing, regardless of the sex of the mounting horse, and part of normal sexual development. Males and females alike are curious about sex and will practise so as to be prepared for the real thing later on. In adult horses, non-reproductive mounting is actually a way of asserting and establishing dominance relationships within the herd. These relationships are essential, because if everybody knows his or her place in the group the herd as a whole will be stronger and more settled, and can spend more time on the vital activities of eating and avoiding predators. The non-sexual nature of this kind of mounting is clear when we consider that an adult mare mounting another will do so regardless of the stage her own reproductive cycle is in.

When one horse repeatedly mounts another, this shows that the dominance contest is not settled. The mounting horse wants to be more dominant but isn't yet sure that he has achieved his goal, so has to keep on asserting himself. His state of mind is similar to that of somebody promoted to a management job but who is not yet sure that other people recognise her new status. She makes a point of showing that she is in charge for a time, then once she feels accepted as manager she will usually relax and be more herself. The horse will be the same. Once the contest is won in his mind he will be able to assert himself in more indirect ways, by a look or a gesture.

Sometimes, as with dominance mounting, horses can be quite

boisterous in their interactions with each other. In general, however, they are careful not to injure each other, because in the wild a horse with even a minor injury ends up targeted by predators. There is usually no need to separate horses engaged in this kind of behaviour, and it is enough to keep an eye on the situation and wait for things to settle down. Having said this, problems can happen if the horses are trying to live out their natural behaviour in an unnatural space. The contest can spiral out of control and lead to injury if the mounting happens in a confined space or if there is only limited access to food or water. The best answer to this problem would be to change the horses' living conditions.

- ∩ A fundamental lack of self-confidence can lead physically dominant horses to assert themselves unnecessarily. The remedy for this would be Larch.

- ∩ Natural leaders can use inappropriate force if they feel their position is under threat. Vine may help this.

- ∩ If dominance contests do get out of control, remember that the horses do not want to hurt each other and are probably frightened themselves. Cherry Plum is the natural remedy to consider at this point.

Feeding problems

Wild horses don't carry or drag burdens. They don't run long distances at top speed. They spend a large part of every day grazing so as to get enough green stuff through their relatively small stomachs. In contrast, we ask horses to carry us and to run further and faster than they would usually choose to, and in so doing use up time they would normally spend grazing. To make up for all these unnatural demands on their strength, time and energy, horses need to eat some unnatural foods if they are going to keep up their fitness and energy levels.

This is true as far as it goes. But it's a mistake to think that any human-devised feed system can replace nature entirely. Spending long periods with no food in the belly and nothing to chew on is one reason horses get bored and suffer from digestive problems. They do best if they have access to grass or hay 24 hours a day, and roughage like this should always make up the bulk of their feed. If the horse is kept in a large enough space or in an open-

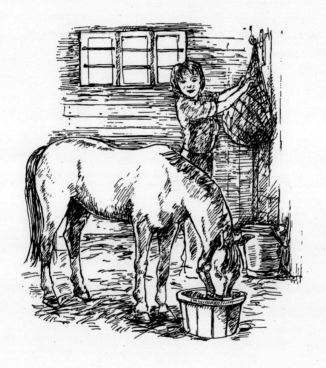

barn system, you can scatter piles of hay in different parts of the barn. Have more piles of hay than there are horses. This allows the horses to eat on the hoof, as they would in the wild, and this has been shown to reduce stress levels. To avoid laminitis, though, be careful about letting horses overfeed on lush grass, and make sure horses sharing an open barn are part of a settled herd.

If horses eat more concentrates than they need for the amount of work they do, then they will put on weight. Your horse may be overweight if you can't see where his ribs end. The answer is to work more or feed less. All adjustments to type or amount of food should be made gradually, and if adjusting the amount of food doesn't have an effect get professional advice on how to address the problem.

Horses lose weight when they are ill or not eating enough food to replace the energy they are using. Your horse may be underweight if you can see each of his ribs and the neck and flanks seem hollow and weak. Possible causes of weight loss include poor teeth, damage to the intestine, worm infestation, liver damage and diarrhoea. Try the obvious things first – worming and increasing the amount of food you are giving – but if this does not help take his temperature to check for fever and ask the vet for a proper diagnosis. If your horse fails to eat for 24 hours treat it as a serious problem and call out the vet at once.

- You might need to treat yourself if your horse is overweight. Do you need Chicory because you are buying love by overfeeding? Or would Red Chestnut help you see that your horse will not starve if you cut down his food intake to the recommended level?

- Walnut will help horses adjust to changes in feed or in feeding regime.

Travel and trailer problems

Horses can be good travellers, but they need time to get used to the idea. That means taking a few short trips in the horse box before you attempt the 100-mile trip to an important competition. It also means that if your horse can't stand getting into his box you will have to help him. Without your patient reassurance, the trailer looks like a dark, dangerous cave, probably full of tigers and bears.

You could try leading him into and out of the box and providing a treat every time he gets in. If you have a trailer with front and rear loading, try leaving it in his field with all the doors open so he can see for himself there is nothing in there. You might even leave his hay ration on the ramp for a few days to get him used to the smell. Gradually work up to a short drive a few yards up the road. As with all retraining, the key is to build up slowly and go back to the previous stage if there is any kind of set-back. See the section on learning on page 79 for more ideas. And remember that horses are big, strong animals. Get professional help if you are not 100 per cent confident of your ability to load and unload a horse safely.

The following remedies can be used to help horses cope with trailer and travel anxieties.

- ∩ Scleranthus has been found to be useful for nausea while travelling.

- ∩ Mimulus will help deal with any specific anxieties to do with getting into the horse box.

- ∩ If you suspect that your horse's fears are due to his having been mistreated in the past, try Star of Bethlehem.

- ∩ Where a horse loses control completely and panics or works himself into a frenzy, consider Rock Rose or Cherry Plum, or give Rescue™ Remedy, which contains both.

- ∩ Walnut can be helpful when horses are upset by new experiences.

- ∩ Try Chestnut Bud if you are having to retrain a horse to accept occasional journeys and you find he is particularly slow to learn.

- ∩ Your driving needs to be smooth and unhurried when you are transporting horses. If this doesn't come easily to you, take some Impatiens.

Boredom

It's hard to imagine that boredom was a big problem when humans lived as hunter – gatherers and every day was a struggle to survive. It's only recently that large numbers of people have been able to replace the day-long job of getting shelter and food with central heating and ten minutes in a supermarket. Civilisation has opened up spaces in our timetable. To fill them up we travel, join clubs, go out dancing and drinking, read books, learn to play the piano, watch television, etc. We demand novelty. To most casual riders our horses are just one more element in a full and exciting life.

Horses have also reaped some of the rewards of civilisation. They have plenty to eat, the best medical care, warm blankets, and – if they only knew it – no need to worry about tigers. By doing all this for them we have opened up space in their timetables too. Unfortunately, large numbers of horses have no opportunity to do exciting things in their new-found spare time. As a result, the average stabled horse lives a life of unrelenting boredom and routine. Everything is done at the same time every day, and the horse has little opportunity to play or express himself or investigate his surroundings. Long-term boredom is recognised as a potent stress factor, and its effects on a horse's mental and physical health can be profound. Research has shown that animals who live boring, understimulated lives are slower to learn, get sick more often, and suffer a range of nutritional and digestive problems. Their ability to relate socially and sexually to other horses also declines.

Imagine living like a stabled horse. You spend most of every day in a small space barely big enough to walk around in. You are alone and have nothing to occupy you, but there is a window, so you spend large parts of the day looking out of it hoping something will happen. You have no control over your life and rely entirely on outside events to give you something to look forward to. The regular highlights of your day are being groomed, being fed, and of course a couple of hours' relative freedom in a field. If you want to go further you can experience this kind of life for real. All you have to do is get yourself locked up in a particularly repressive and old-fashioned prison. For human prisoners also look forward to the few regular events that break up the day – the exercise yard, dinner time and the shower room – and know exactly what should happen and when. If there is some break in the routine, then trapped humans, like trapped horses, get upset and unruly.

Because equine prisoners get upset when their longed-for feed or grooming session doesn't arrive on time, people have come to believe that horses are creatures of habit and that an unvarying routine is the only way to manage them. This is simply not true. Horses are no more addicted to boredom than we are. They thrive best if their lives are interesting, varied and full of things to do and think about. They like to be able to make choices about where they go and when. On hot days, the free herd decides to graze high and exposed areas, where they can keep a good lookout and have the benefit of any breezes that are blowing. On wet and windy days, they move lower down and look for sheltered areas. The poor stabled horse tries to make choices as best he can, and stands at the back of his box in wet weather, or at the window when it is fine. But it is a pathetic substitute for real life.

The answer to your horse's boredom is to make his life less

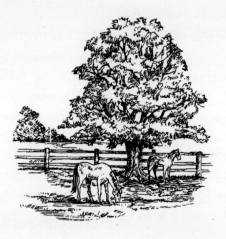

boring. First, make sure he is turned out with his pair-bond as much as possible. If possible, the pair should be turned out as part of a settled herd. In the summer 24-hours-a-day turn-out is the ideal as long as there is some shade and shelter available. If your yard can only manage three hours a day or so, or can't commit to turning him out every day, change yards. And look at the areas where turn-out happens. Is the paddock flat, square and boring? Or are there slopes, hills and trees, places to play and places to find shelter?

When your horse has to be in a stable don't lock him in. It's better to fence off an area in front of the stable – the bigger the better – and leave the door open. This at least gives him the chance to decide for himself if he wants to be in or out, and he can see much more of the world and so feel more comfortable in his environment. If he has been kept inside for a very long time he may take time to adjust to the idea that he can go out. Some stabled horses even develop agoraphobia. But most will welcome the new freedom and will choose to stay outside except in very bad weather.

A second area where you can make life more interesting is food. In the wild, horses look for variety and enjoy looking for different sorts of grass, fruits and vegetables. They may spend up to ten per cent of their time eating leaves, budding twigs and bark off trees. They move around while eating, and eat when they want to, as many as 16 hours out of 24, and at all times of the day and night.

As far as possible, you should aim to give your horse the freedom to do the same as he would in the wild. Provide hay 24 hours a day, and provide variety by hanging half a dozen different fruits and vegetables from the stable roof. Use different lengths of string to make things more interesting and give him something to think about. Bring tree branches for him to chew on, or even small logs, after checking with the vet that the species of tree is not poisonous to horses (see also page 171). Try scattering concentrate around the stable or mixing it in with his piles of hay, so that he can eat

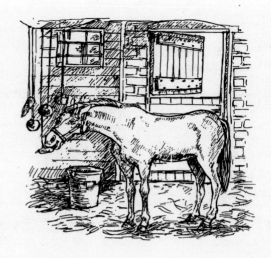

on the hoof. This will also mean he has to do some work to get his food, and because mealtimes will take longer he will be more occupied for more of the time. Feed smaller amount more often – four meals a day is good, and six is better – and if possible give some of them during the night. And don't let feed times become a routine – feed at different times so that he does not fall into the habit of spending time thinking about the next meal.

With a good rider aboard, most horses enjoy hacking. The experience can be made even more interesting if you put some thought into where you go and how you manage your horse. Where possible try to vary the route and the times of day – just like us, horses enjoy seeing the countryside looking different in the morning from the way it looks in the late afternoon. Provided the hack is safe for horses you could take advantage of his natural ability to find his way back to home territory, and let him choose the route when you turn for home. He may be a bit confused if you suddenly do this after years of taking the decision yourself, but after the first few times he will get the idea and enjoy the challenge. Finally, you could upgrade your own riding skills by taking a course in Parelli Natural Horsemanship or one of the other natural training systems. This will show you safe ways to allow your horse to take more decisions for himself, and this is the best long-term cure for boredom. See the back of this book for some useful addresses.

∩ Horses may seem to give up when they are bored. Remedies that could help include Wild Rose for resigned acceptance, Gorse if he seems resigned and depressed, Hornbeam if he seems to lack get-up-and-go, and Clematis if he escapes by sleeping more than usual.

∩ Frustration when routines are disrupted could be helped by Vervain or Willow, depending on how personally he seems to take the disruption and how vocal he is about protesting.

Depression

Horses get depressed for different reasons, just like we do. Sometimes the cause is physical – illness, injury or pain – so as a precaution call out the vet if your horse seems unhappy or troubled. Other types of depression are caused by events in the horse's life, such as a companion dying or going away, or by living conditions. Stabled horses may suffer from depression when a lack of stimulation leads to listlessness, loss of appetite and stereotypical behaviour (see page 106), while lack of shelter can cause depression in outdoor horses.

A third type of depression comes from within the horse's mind and doesn't seem to be related to any obvious physical or environmental problem. This can be the most difficult to treat using orthodox methods, because lifestyle changes and physical check-ups will not help, while medication just suppresses the problem and can cause side effects. Fortunately the remedies include a number of treatment options for depression, and with care it is usually possible to help the horse to regain his emotional equilibrium.

- Gentian where the horse seems a little despondent due to something going wrong – for example not getting an expected treat, or not going down a favourite path – and just needs a little encouragement.

- Gorse where he seems to have given up and adopted a pessimistic attitude. There seems no hope, even though there might be possible solutions to hand.

- Mustard where there seems no reason for his unhappiness.

- Willow if he seems to be wallowing in unhappiness and getting a perverse pleasure from sulking and grumbling.

- Where there is serious illness or the horse is near death or suffering extreme anguish, then Sweet Chestnut may bring some relief.

Displacement behaviour

Next time you see television coverage of an awards ceremony or the opening night of a film, pay special attention. In particular, look at what the celebrities do when they first get out of their cars and start walking through the gap left in the mass of photographers and fans to right and left. Nine times out of ten they will make some small and unnecessary gesture with their hands, such as smoothing back their already smooth hair, or brushing down an immaculate lapel, or straightening freshly pressed shirt cuffs. These small gestures are displacement behaviours.

A displacement behaviour is something that we do when we are under stress but can't do the thing we would like to do. Facing the flashbulbs and the hysterical screams is daunting. Perhaps the celebrity wants to turn and run or get back in the car and hide. But she can't do that, so her brain satisfies her need to do something by triggering another action instead. This brings her a measure of relief and comfort, enough to get her across the carpet and into the theatre. Triggers for displacement behaviours in people include fear, frustration and confusion. Related displacement activities include yawning when nervous, drumming fingers or jiggling legs when frustrated, and scratching our heads when confused.

All mammals display displacement behaviours – chimpanzees actually scratch their heads when puzzled just like we do. You have probably seen horses performing displacement activities many times without realising it. For example, a horse who has been put into a field next door to where his herd is will often run up and down the fence and call out to the other horses. This is natural and you can see why he is doing it. But sometimes he feels so frustrated that he stops running and performs other movements – head tossing and foreleg raising. This is displacement behaviour. Perhaps you were grooming your horse ready for a competition, or picking out his feet, or loading him into the trailer, when he began to yawn. He wasn't tired or bored, just nervous. Or maybe he shook a foreleg at you when you first tried to fit a halter on him. He wasn't threatening you, he was just confused about your intentions. Or maybe you have caught him chewing his lead rope, or grabbing onto or biting through his bit, or mouthing the grooming kit, or rolling when you lead him, or grabbing mouthfuls of grass when another horse comes up to him. Some horses will even give themselves a quick nip, in the same way we might bite our lips or wring our hands until they hurt. If he could have he might have run away, but instead he did something else as a way of destressing himself. These behaviours were just his way of getting through the day-to-day stresses of living.

It's easy for us to misinterpret displacement behaviours because they do not always have the same meaning. We may assume that a horse raising his foreleg at the farrier is being aggressive and getting ready to strike out. But he may just be frustrated at being tied up, or frightened and wanting to move away. The same gesture when you are trying to teach him something could simply mean that he is confused and unsure of what you want. Having to wait for feed is one common reason why a horse will paw the ground with frustration – his jaws are ready to move but you are taking your time about feeding him. But he may do the same thing if you are standing closer to him than he would like, or you are too near his feed and he is worried that you will take it away again.

The identification problem is made worse because many apparent displacement behaviours have other causes. A horse who raises his leg may be injured or in pain. Horses who bite themselves to excess may be severely disturbed and need help. Pawing can be so prolonged and vigorous that it wears down the horse's hoof and damages the stable floor, a phenomenon that suggests the horse is severely depressed. A good equine vet should be able to spot serious problems like these. Always call one in if you are not sure what is happening.

If your horse tends to use displacement behaviour a lot he could be unhappy, confused, dissatisfied or just plain frightened. Using physical means to curb the behaviour, such as replacing rubber bits with metal ones so he can't chew through them, will not stop him feeling this way. The real answer must be to improve the situation for him. A combination of remedies and behaviour and environmental modification techniques can help to achieve this.

The first thing to do is to see if the displacement behaviour is associated with any particular cause. If your horse chews on the lead rope when you are grooming him, he is probably frustrated because he wants to groom you in return but is unable to. If he rolls when you lead him forward, the cause is probably fear of leaving the herd and/or anxiety at being led into an unfamiliar or threatening space. If he snatches up grass when other horses come near, he has a fear of being approached. In other cases, however, the cause can be hard to define, and you may need to call in a behaviourist to help you identify what the problem is.

The next step is to change things around so as to minimise your horse's stress levels. Often this means removing causes of frustration, and using habituation techniques (see page 80) to help him see that there is no danger in the situation. This will help him relax. And of course, positively reinforce him when he does what you want.

Following this principle, you might help the lead-chewing horse by giving him something else to play with when you groom him. If he can 'groom' a toy while being groomed, he will not feel frustrated, and you in turn will go through fewer lead ropes. If he paws at the ground before every feed time, try changing the

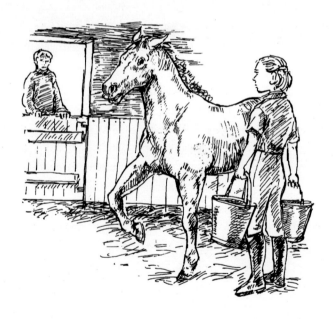

feeding routine. Feed frequently and at different times, and don't create a ritual that tells him when to get excited. You might even prepare the feed the night before to avoid the peak of excitement when he can hear it being prepared but can't yet get to it. If he paws even when he has his food, try leaving him alone to eat it in peace so that he will get used to the idea that he doesn't have to be on guard all the time when eating. Once he has got used to eating alone, start to reintroduce yourself in a non-threatening and indirect manner. Try talking to a friend outside the stable and out of sight while he eats, or opening the door but not going in, or being visible at a distance and busy with something else. If he tends to paw when the vet or farrier is working on him, look for ways of improving his general level of confidence. Get friends of yours to lead him around, pick out his feet and so on. If the farrier is the only male human he ever sees, get some other male friends involved so that he associates men with pleasant things like being fed and exercised. If the vet always wears white overalls, get some yourself and wear them. Get him used to being handled and touched and examined in non-threatening situations.

- ∩ Walnut is known as the link breaker, and can help horses leave old habits behind. It is also good as protection against outside influences in general.

- ∩ General lack of confidence usually indicates Mimulus or Larch or both.

- ∩ Mimulus is for straightforward fears in horses, such as his anxious thought that somebody might take his food away.

- ∩ Confusion in a horse could indicate any of a number of remedies – start by looking up Scleranthus, Cerato, White Chestnut and Gentian.

- ∩ Crab Apple can help cleanse repetitive mannerisms and obsessive – compulsive movements.

Stereotypical behaviour

Stereotypical behaviour is the name psychologists give to apparently purposeless behaviours that repeat over and over without any variation. We see them in very disturbed children, who may rock back and forth or bang walls. Compulsive hand-washing is another human manifestation of something that is associated with mental illness, trauma and severe depression. We see them too in zoo animals: tigers pacing the same route up and down their cages for hours on end, gorillas hunched in a corner picking endlessly at the same patch of fur.

Behaviourists recognise many kinds of stereotypical behaviour in horses. Three of the most common are crib-biting, in which the horse bites into a wooden surface and arches his neck; wind-sucking; and weaving, which involves rocking from side to side. Horses often hang their heads over the stable door while they weave. Even 'normal' behaviour such as head tossing, eating bedding, pawing and walking around can become compulsive.

Warmer-blooded breeds are especially inclined to develop stereotypical behaviours. Upbringing and training may also have an impact, as may artificial diets. In the wild, horses spend as many as 16 hours a day grazing, but concentrated feeds are quickly consumed and leave the horse at a loose end when his instincts tell him that he should be feeding. Gnawing wood and wind-sucking may be one way of relieving the compulsion to feed.

If feeding is the whole problem a constant supply of hay will help it. But the main cause of stereotypical behaviour is being kept in a stable. Indeed, stereotypical behaviour is almost unknown in horses that have not spent at least part of their lives stabled. These apparently motiveless acts are the horse's way of expressing long-term depression, unbearable boredom, tension and stress. Preventing crib-biting by fitting metal caps to woodwork or painting on foul-tasting substances, or fitting metal bars to stable openings to stop horses from weaving, or having recourse to surgery to prevent head tossing, does *not* cure the problem, any more than tying a suicidal human to a post would cure her mental disturbance. These so-called solutions are extremely cruel and can only make the horse's suffering worse.

The only humane answer to stereotypical behaviour is to make your horse's life more bearable by providing as natural an environment as possible. He should not be locked away and should not be kept in solitary confinement. He should live outdoors with others of his kind. If this isn't possible, make sure he gets turned out at least once a day, and that he doesn't have to live alone in traditional stabling. If he socialises well and is already part of an established herd then an open-plan barn of the type advocated by the Natural Animal Centre in England is a better type of shelter when he simply has to be inside. If it is impossible to keep other horses or provide an open barn you can still provide some permanent company in the form of a goat or sheep. And you can make the stable environment more interesting by giving him toys to play with. Anything with an interesting shape will do, as long as the horse can pick it up and won't choke on it.

For more ideas on improving your horse's living arrangements, see page 153. Remember that your vet can refer you to a qualified behaviourist if you need help with a distressed horse. And you can start to use gentle forms of complementary medicines right away to try to help his state of mind.

- Crab Apple is the main remedy for compulsive behaviours, but it can't help if the living conditions causing the behaviour are not addressed at the same time.

- Animals going into a new scheme of life can take time to adjust, even if the changes are beneficial. Walnut will help them adjust to change, and also help break old habits like crib-biting, which may continue even after you give them freedom and a chance to build relationships in a herd.

Hyperactivity

The horse's body clock is set differently from ours. Horses only sleep about three hours out of 24, and when they do sleep it is in five-minute snatches. They lie down where possible, but because of the danger of being eaten they will only do so if they feel especially safe. Sick horses may refuse to lie down at all because of the difficulty they would have getting up in a hurry.

To us the horse's normal behaviour can look like hyperactivity. But true hyperactivity is a different matter. It is characterised by extreme alertness and activity. There may be aggressive or irritable behaviour, or the horse may develop stereotypical behaviours (see the previous section). Sometimes hyperactivity is chronic, and sometimes it emerges only when the horse is under particular stress.

Allergies are one known cause of hyperactivity. Others include lack of exercise, overfeeding of heating foods, and loneliness.

Your vet can help you check for allergies. The need for exercise may mean a complete change in turn-out routine – 24-hours-a-day turn-out is the ideal in all but the harshest winters. Make sure too that your horse has access to grazing or hay around the clock. Grazing should form the bulk of his diet even if he needs some concentrates to keep up with his workload. Which leaves the problem of loneliness.

Horses who don't have regular company find it hard to relax because they feel obliged to keep a lookout for danger all the time. They don't learn how to communicate with other horses, so they are forced to play by themselves, bucking and kicking out even when there are other horses around. The real cure for this problem is to turn your horse out in an established herd, or at least provide him with a pair-bond. This lets him share lookout duties so that he can get some real rest, and allows a natural outlet for social needs. (See 'Meeting a new pair-bond' on page 160 if you want to find a pair-bond for your horse.)

○ Where stress is causing hyperactivity, define the stress and select the appropriate remedies. Common remedies include Mimulus to deal with fear and anxiety, Star of Bethlehem for shock, White Chestnut for worrying thoughts, and Walnut to help adjust to changes.

○ Horses who are overenthusiastic about the things they like and never switch off can be helped with Vervain. Another possibility is Impatiens – these horses will rush from one thing to another and get bored quickly.

○ Irritable, aggressive horses might need Beech or Vine.

○ Crab Apple is the remedy for obsessive, repetitive behaviour – but see also the section on stereotypical behaviour, page 106.

Fear and anxiety

Some fears are natural to the horse. Claustrophobia is a life-preserving reaction in any animal that needs open space to escape from predators. Loneliness produces anxiety in any herd animal. And if you have fragile legs it's natural to get very nervous at anything that might threaten them, such as unfamiliar paths, water and boggy ground. Horses are happier in a crocodile because they have the assurance that another horse has already tried the ground and found it passable.

All prey animals are especially sensitive to painful and anxiety-producing experiences because their next mistake always threatens to be their last. Avoiding a situation that has placed them in trouble in the past is an obvious and intelligent reaction. This is why horses develop aversions to particular situations, people and places – one bad event leaves its mark and anything associated with that event is best avoided in future. Unexpected alterations can unnerve them as well, at least until they have had a chance to check things out to be sure there is no danger involved. Even a freshly painted fence may be a worry. This explains the occasional reluctance to do something quite normal, such as turning into a familiar lane. Perhaps someone's radio is playing, or a usually open window is curtained, or you are in a particular hurry. To the horse, these additions to the environment could signal some unexpected threat, so he will want to go cautiously.

Some particularly anxious horses seem to inherit fearfulness in the same way they inherit coat colour and conformation. Other fears go back to the first few days of life, so young foals who do not have regular and reassuring contact with humans may grow up into wary adults, reluctant to trust people without a lot of patience and coaxing. Dealing with fears like this can take a lot of time and patience. Other fears are contingent, such as nervous reactions to passing traffic and dogs, or the close attentions of a vet. Simple training techniques can be used to get a horse used to these things. (See page 79 for more on how horses learn.)

Anxiety is a common cause of many apparently unrelated behavioural problems, including backing up, running away or running back home, refusing to go forwards and rearing. Horses who seem depressed or upset or aggressive are often in a state of fear. In the case of aggression, it's worth remembering that people eat animals like horses – or have done in the past – so any horse unsure of our intentions is likely to feel afraid. Fear is by far the most common cause of aggression towards humans. Even the most reserved and mild horse will eventually kick out if he is frightened enough and can't find a way to escape.

The remedies can be an enormous help in relieving fear. More centred in himself, a more calm and secure horse will also make a quicker and fuller recovery from illness and injury. If you do have trouble or feel out of your depth, seek professional advice and ask your vet to refer you to a qualified animal behaviourist.

- Choose Mimulus if the anxiety has a definite cause, such as dogs or traffic. Where possible, take steps to habituate the horse to the fearful thing, and make sure you are not sending anxiety signals yourself, such as tensing up and changing your seat whenever a lorry approaches on a road. Mimulus also applies if the horse seems to be a shy and nervous type in general.

- Try Aspen if there is no reason for the fear. Some stabled horses develop agoraphobia if they are suddenly turned out to graze, especially if they are by themselves. Their illogical fear that 'something' might happen may be an indicator for trying Aspen first.

- Select Red Chestnut if you feel that the horse is overly anxious about the welfare of a pair-bond or foal.

- Choose Cherry Plum for loss of control and irrational and sometimes violent acts. A horse in this state loses his ability to control his actions, and may strike out at you or even injure himself. Horses in this state are frightened by their own loss of control as much as anything: think of a toddler having a tantrum and screaming with a mix of rage and fright, and that is Cherry Plum.

- Select Rock Rose for absolute terror. A horse in a Rock Rose state will be so frightened of something that he may bolt. If he can't escape he may freeze where he is and be unable to do anything.

- As a quick fix you can give Rescue™ Remedy to calm things down, but try to select one or a mix of the single remedies if the problem is chronic.

Kinds of fear: horses and pigs

A we saw in the last section, fear is a core emotion in horses. As prey animals they are wired to be especially alert to anything that could pose a threat. This is why so many things make them anxious, from horse boxes to plastic bags to tractors – the rustle of a bag caught in a hedge is very similar to the noise a tiger might make stepping through leaves. Better to not take a chance, and get away at once. But of all the fears that horses have, fear of pigs is one of the strongest. And dealing with it – and with another common kind of fear, separation anxiety – will give us a good opportunity to outline skills that can be used to help horses deal with many different types of fear.

Many horses live on or near farms of one sort or another. They may be nervous of cows, sheep and other farm animals, but nothing else provokes the extreme panic of a horse who has caught sight of a pig. If we want to understand their feelings we could start by looking for a similar pattern in humans. We are not usually frightened of pigs, but many of us panic when we see a snake or spider. Just seeing one in a film can be enough for some people to feel they want to leave the room or close their eyes in terror. Even tiny children can display this behaviour, without any obvious learning having taken place. Is there a mechanism that would explain these fears in both horses and humans?

It turns out that there is, and it lies in the theory of *preparedness*. According to biologists, part of being born human or equine (or anything else) is to have particular tendencies pre-programmed into the brain. This means that an animal is already inclined to take a particular view of a new object or experience even before encountering it for the first time. We (and other animals) do this by associating its shape or movement with a potential outcome. Some spider bites are poisonous and can kill. According to the preparedness theory, a human faced with something spider-shaped associates it with the outcome of being bitten, and this is why fear of spiders is so common among people.

Pigs aren't carnivores in the sense of hunting horses. They will scavenge off dead animals but this in itself poses no threat to a live horse. But male pigs do carry weapons for use in the wild, and they can be formidable. The sharp tusks of a wild boar are capable of killing an animal who threatens the boar or his family. And we know that millions of years ago horses were much smaller than they are now, so that a horse disturbing a boar unexpectedly would have had to face a very dangerous opponent. In an evolutionary sense, then, horses' fears make at least as much sense as our own fear of snakes. (And the theory also explains why animals who eat snakes, like secretary birds and mongooses, are not frightened of them in the same way that other animals are – they associate them with a full belly.)

If we accept that horses feel about pigs much as we feel about snakes, we already have a clearer idea of how they feel. It is an irrational fear, in the sense that it may be out of proportion, but just as it does no good to tell somebody afraid of spiders not to be silly, so it will not help to treat the horse as silly or stupid if he is scared of pigs. The fear is real, and must be treated as such.

In the past, one way of 'curing' horses of their fear of pigs was to put a pig and a horse in an enclosed space together and leave them alone to get on with it. The technical term for this approach is *flooding*. The theory behind flooding is that eventually the horse will stop panicking and realise that he is not going to get hurt, and in this way he will lose his fear. However, there are a number of reasons why we should never use flooding with horses. First, there is a real danger that the horse or the pig or both will be injured. The horse may kick out at the pig in his terror, or he may try to get over a fence or break down a stable door. Second, the intense distress felt by the horse (and by the poor pig, who will pick up on the horse's panic) is cruel in its own right. (Being locked in a small space with the thing that you most fear was precisely the form of torture used in Room 101.) Third, there is a chance that it will actually *sensitise* the horse to pigs so that he is even more terrified of them in the future than he was in the past. Fourth, even in the cases where flooding works, the loss of fear may reverse at any time – i.e. the cure may not last very long.

It is safer and much more effective to manage the horse's encounter with pigs so as to make it gradual and positive and cause as little stress as possible. This means using habituation (see page 80). This will certainly take longer than flooding, but the results will be better. As to exactly how long it will take, this depends on the horse's breed, his past experiences, general state of health, reproductive status and on what he is like as an individual.

To see how habituation works in practice, here is what happened at the Natural Animal Centre when it was decided to introduce the horses to some piglets. The first step was to put the piglets into a field next to the horses. Both fields were large enough to allow the animals to move away to a safe distance from each other

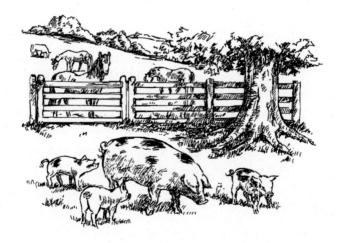

whenever they wanted, and there was a strong fence between them. After several weeks, even the most nervy of the horses had got used to the presence of the pigs in the next field and was back to behaving in a calm and settled way.

This achieved, the gate in the fence was opened and the pigs were able to go into the horses' field. Most of the horses remained calm. They had already habituated to the pigs and there was no trouble. However, one or two individuals tried to get close to the pigs and stamp on them. (This is natural behaviour in a horse when there is something strange but not particularly threatening in the area – this is why they paw at footballs and other new toys.) The horses who behaved like this needed more time to get used to the pigs and accept them as part of the scenery. Accordingly, they were further habituated to the piglets in a variety of situations for several more weeks, and in circumstances that placed the piglets out of danger. For example, the horse might be brought into the yard for grooming, with the pigs penned in nearby. Over time, even the most jumpy of the horses accepted the pigs and no longer reacted when they were present. As a result, these horses are now safer to ride, and have been freed of an unnecessary fear.

Kinds of fear: separation anxiety

Separation anxiety is a well-known problem in the dog world. It's a fear of abandonment, and happens when a dog's owner leaves him alone without having prepared him in advance. In their anxiety to escape and find their owner, dogs have been known to gnaw their way through walls and metal doors; more common reactions are tearing up curtains and chewing shoes.

Strictly speaking separation anxiety is about the relationship between an animal and a human being. Horses do not readily form such strong bonds with individual humans, at least not in the same way that dogs do, but they do form strong attachments to the herd and in particular to their pair-bond. Horses who become agitated when their pair-bond is removed, or nap towards the yard, or will only get into a trailer if pair-bond goes too, are all behaving in ways analogous to the anxious dog, and the root cause is the same: feeling abandoned.

As we might expect, the more nervy breeds of horses – warm- and hot-bloods – are genetically more inclined to suffer from separation anxiety. There is also evidence that upbringing has an effect. Horses reared by themselves are at greater risk, as are those who only have limited opportunities for socialising. And once the problem begins it tends to get worse. At first your horse may only seem a little bit anxious when his pair-bond leaves, but without early help clear symptoms will soon emerge. These include profuse sweating, defecation, and an inability to eat or drink when he is by himself. Other behaviours associated with this condition are standing stock still at the gate, whinnying with the head held high, and agitated running along the fenceline. The latter may start quite sedately, with the horse only walking up and down, but as the problem gets worse so he will trot and then canter, and his head will come up and toss.

Unfortunately, the cure for separation anxiety is not as simple as sticking another horse in the field along with the first one. The problem is more tightly focused: the horse is anxious about being apart from *one particular horse*. We can see this clearly when we look at horses who live in herds. Remove an anxious horse's pair-bond and he will display symptoms of separation anxiety even if the rest of the herd is still around him. The symptoms stop when the pair-bond comes back. At the risk of anthropomorphism, we could liken the horse's feelings to our own if we were to lose sight of our partner in a crowd. The crowd is no comfort – it's our partner that we miss.

Separation anxiety is easier to avoid than to cure, and this applies especially if you are buying a thoroughbred or an Arab or one of the other warmer-blooded breeds. We can start when we first buy a horse, by refusing to deal with studs that rear horses in solitary confinement. If everyone did this these yards would go out of business and there would be fewer anxious and depressed horses in the world. We should only deal with studs that allow horses to mix with others, and live as natural a life as possible. Horses who grow up in good environments get used to the idea that other horses come and go from time to time, and that there is no reason to worry about this.

If you already have a horse who is showing signs of separation anxiety you can still help him deal with his anxiety better. To do this you can use counter-conditioning to teach him that being apart from his pair-bond is not a cause for concern. As with all training, you need to go very slowly and repeat often. Start by going into the field and catching the horse's pair-bond. Put her head collar on, then let her go immediately. In severe cases, the simple fact of your catching his pair-bond will be enough to set off symptomatic anxiety behaviour in the anxious horse. In any case, you can't progress until he is used to seeing you catching, collaring and releasing his pair-bond, and has learned that this process by itself is not a cause for concern. Do it several times a day then, and be prepared to repeat over a period of weeks.

When you are able to go through the collaring process without him getting anxious, then you can move on to the next step. Having caught the pair-bond, lead her through the gate and then immediately return her to the field and let her go. At first this may make the first horse anxious: he accepts that collaring is not always a problem, but he has yet to accept that actually leaving the field is OK. So you must repeat the process several times a day until he understands that his pair-bond always comes back, and he shows no sign of anxiety.

The final stage of the process is to begin to separate the horses. At first you should only do this for a few minutes at a time, and allow them to see and reach each other across the fence. Once the anxious horse accepts this you can start to move his pair-bond further away. If at any point he starts to become anxious, that means you are trying to go too fast. Again, it may take weeks of daily repetition before you can actually lead the pair-bond completely out of his sight. And you may also find that his anxiety is context-specific, so that having got him used to separation in his usual field you may need to repeat the whole process to get him used to separation in the yard, entering a trailer by himself, and so on.

There are no short cuts to dealing with this problem, and people who advocate tearing the horses apart in one fell swoop are wrong – for sentimental reasons, yes, in that it is extremely cruel, but also for hard scientific reasons. Abrupt separation does not work in the long term, because even if the horse seems to resign himself to the situation he will still, and for ever more, be liable to fall back into a state of uncontrolled anxiety at any time.

You can get help if your horse suffers from this problem. The vet will be able to prescribe tranquillisers, which can help keep him calm while you use training techniques like those outlined here to help him overcome his anxiety. She will also be able to refer your horse to a qualified behaviourist if you need expert help. And of course complementary therapies can be very helpful, including carefully-chosen remedies.

∩ The nearest equivalent to a tranquilliser – and far more gentle – would be to give doses of Rescue™ Remedy to help keep the anxious horse calm during the process of counter-conditioning.

∩ The basic fear remedy for this kind of situation is Mimulus. Red Chestnut may apply for horses whose fear centres more around the welfare of the departing pair-bond. Rock Rose will help genuine panic.

∩ Chicory is helpful for separated horses who are usually very affectionate with their pair-bonds, and find even short absences difficult to deal with. Others who insist on having company but are not especially affectionate may do better on Heather.

Aggression

Horses are big and strong. If your horse starts barging into or chasing you it can be a frightening experience. And it can be worrying to see one of your horses kicking out at another or biting. But it's not enough in these circumstances to label the aggressive horse as 'difficult' or 'dangerous'. Instead we need to understand the reason for his behaviour.

All animals show aggression in some circumstances. This is normal, and not something to be avoided. As the behaviourist, Konrad Lorenz, showed in the 1960s, aggression helps species to survive. Among other benefits, it keeps animals a certain distance away from each other, so helping them spread across available living space. It ensures that those best able to survive will breed and so pass on their genes to later generations. And it establishes a pecking order that allows the establishment of a stable social order. All of these benefits are enjoyed by horses in the wild: herds are settled societies; they stay apart from each other so as not compete for the same resources, and the strongest and brightest individuals lead the herds and get to breed most often. Unfortunately, however, the way we ask horses to live does not always allow behaviour to develop naturally. This can lead too often to genuine problems with aggression, sometimes at an intensity that is out of proportion with the situation.

The actions we can take to manage aggression depend on the kind of aggression that is being displayed. In all cases the first thing to do is to invite the vet to check the horse to be sure that undiagnosed pain or some other physical cause is not the reason for the behaviour. For example, older horses can develop arthritis, which may make them especially irritable when younger horses hurt them by playing or grooming too vigorously.

Horses inherit a predisposition to aggression from their parents, and the more reactive breeds are quicker to show aggression than cold-bloods. But however hot-blooded the horse, there is always

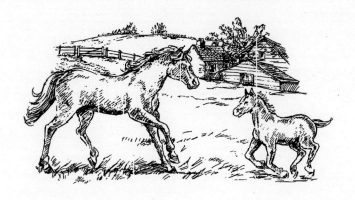

a *reason* for aggressive behaviour. For example, maternal aggression, as the name implies, is mostly associated with mares protecting their foals. You can reduce this kind of aggression by reducing the mare's anxiety. One way to do this is to let her and her foal share a field with other mares and foals so that they can all watch out for each other, as they would in the wild. But maternal aggression can also kick in when the mare is in season, as a result of hormonal changes. If you suspect this you will need to ask the vet to confirm the diagnosis and possibly suggest a course of treatment. Mares who tend to be anxious with people at the best of times may become overtly aggressive once they have a foal at foot. For this reason there is a strong argument for not allowing poorly socialised mares to breed at all. Why bring more nervous horses into an already crowded world?

Fear aggression is in general the most common kind of aggression. Usually it starts when a horse feels threatened and is unable to get out of range. For example, two horses might be playing when one of them decides he has had enough and wants to move away. If they are in a small field and he can't escape the attentions of his erstwhile playmate he may become fearful and start biting or kicking to try to stop the game. If your horse seems especially nervous and inclined towards fear aggression you could try removing him from the herd for a time and pair-bonding him with another horse who is confident and very relaxed. Once they have teamed up they can be reintroduced to the herd, with the hope that the calming influence of the second horse will help the first find his feet better.

A particular form of fear aggression occurs when a horse is afraid that he will lose his food. This leads him to guard his food and try to stop others approaching it. The answer to this is to find him an area where he can eat by himself without feeling under pressure from other horses entering his space.

Another common occasion for aggression between horses is herd definition: the coming together of a new group, for example, or the job of teaching wayward youngsters their place, or assimilating a new addition into an existing group. We may see a number of fights break out in a new herd, or see a newcomer chased away every time he comes near an established herd. The reason for this aggression is a mix of territorial aggression and dominance aggression, arguments over the herd pecking order. On the one hand, it is normal for the herd to defend its territory against an intruder and for each individual in the herd to defend his own personal space. On the other hand, some horses in the herd may feel that their personal ranking in the hand is threatened by the new horse, especially if the newcomer is similar to them in terms of size and strength and age.

As herd animals, horses are inclined to cooperate with each other. We can often allow dominance aggression problems within established herds to sort themselves out, but only as long as the quarreling horses have enough space to get away from each other. This will allow the subordinate horses to keep out of the way of the more dominant herd members without provoking aggression. New horses should be introduced to the herd slowly and with care, and only at times when the existing pecking order is well-established and working smoothly.

Owners who try to help subordinate horses by giving them treats first, or making a special fuss of them, may only make things worse. The higher-ranking horses may see this as a threat to their position and make their point with more aggression. The risk of making social gaffes like this means that when we interact with the herd we need to be sensitive to relationships within it.

Horses do bully each other sometimes, especially when conditions are hard and the bullies are hungry. Again, you will not solve the problem by trying to 'make it up' to the bullied animal. Instead, the answer is to make sure there is enough food and water in enough locations so that the victim can feed without being pressurised by the bullies, and enough space to run to if the pressure gets too much. Make sure there is an even number of horses in a herd so that the animals can pair up – victims enhance their social status this way, and are more likely to be accepted if they have bonded with an existing herd member. If bullying doesn't stop you may need to introduce the bullied horse into another herd, but this should be a last resort as it may upset the existing social structure in the new herd.

Bullying can be a problem in stables as well, even where bullies can't physically get to their victims, because much of the threatening is done through body language and eye contact. Common sense is a good guide when placing horses in stables, and bullies and their victims should never be stalled next to or opposite each other. Ideally, of course, they should not be in stables at all.

Studying body language can help you decide why your horse feels aggressive. Striking with front legs and biting are offensive movements, while kicking out with rear legs is a defensive reaction. Ears pointing back may mean a readiness to fight, but can also mean that the horse is focusing on something going on behind him, perhaps getting ready to move back and away from something that is making him uneasy, or that he is submitting to another horse. Look at the body position and direction to see which is which – an aggressive horse moves towards the thing he wants to threaten, and may move his head and neck like a snake as he goes, while a threatened horse turns aside.

As we saw when we looked at how to read Equus (see page 55), interpreting behaviour can be difficult. Showing the teeth in a fixed open mouth can be aggressive and indicate a desire to bite, but a horse offering to groom by snapping his teeth together and mouthing is actually trying to appease aggression. Grooming is a friendly behaviour, so if your horse is in the habit of nipping your clothes this may not be aggression, however unwelcome you might find it. Truly aggressive biting tends to be very sudden, and often comes out of the blue. And snaking neck movements and flattened ears are used in play between friendly animals, in much the same way that children enjoy shouting and wrestling with playmates and puppies attack their littermates.

Just as lower-ranked horses avoid dominants in the herd, so a horse's natural reaction when a human approaches is to move away. This reflects our status as a potential predator. But he can't run if he is tied up or locked into a stable, so he has to do something else. If he got used to humans at an early age he will cope with our proximity by fiddling about. But if he views us as a serious threat he may decide his only option is to fight. How do we deal with this?

The obvious answer to an aggressive horse is to get away fast and get a more experienced person to catch him. Unfortunately, this may make things worse. Leaving a field every time your horse charges you tells him that this is a good way to deal with you, because it works. You are reinforcing his behaviour and he is more likely to show aggression next time a similar situation arises. This doesn't mean that you should take risks with your personal safety. Getting out may be the right thing to do in the short term. But in the long term you need a better solution.

If fear is the reason for his aggression, the answer is to spend time alone with him doing things that he likes doing. You want him to associate your presence with good things such as food and grooming. So aim to be with him when he eats – though you may need to do this in a sensitive way and at a distance so as to avoid making him even more nervous. Look at the way in which you approach him, to be sure that you are being as non-threatening as possible. Don't walk into his personal space all in one go, or move suddenly. Let him know you are there first, then pause for time before moving forward slowly and at an angle.

We have already said that pain often causes aggression, and that the vet should be consulted as a matter of course. A good equine dentist will make sure his teeth are well cared for and a saddler will check that his saddle is a good fit. But don't forget to look at other aspects of his management routine. Restricted horses sometimes lash out through frustration, so training him to stand still for grooming is better than tying him up all the time. Don't allow him to become too territorial about his field or barn: be there yourself, have other people visit him, and spend time with him on neutral territory. Some horses may feel inclined to be dominant even over humans, or use painful nipping as a form of play. You can approach these problems by training in Parelli Natural Horsemanship, or one of the other natural management systems, so as to communicate more effectively with your horse. If he nips a lot give him a toy to play with to redirect his attention.

Inevitably you may misread a situation several times before you hit on the right explanation for your horse's aggression. If aggression is serious or causing real problems then you should consider getting professional help. This need not stop you from trying the remedies at once, since selecting by trial and error will at least do no harm. Here are some examples of remedies that might apply.

∩ Mimulus where aggression is caused by fear and you can identify a reason for the fear. Look for aggression towards particular types of people (for example, children, vets, other horses) or in particular situations (at a show, or whenever you take a particular track, for example) as these indicate that the horse may be afraid of something specific.

∩ Star of Bethlehem if the fear is due to some unresolved shock or trauma. For example, a horse who has been beaten in the past may react with fear aggression if he sees someone approaching him holding something. This would call for a mix of Mimulus and Star of Bethlehem.

∩ Cherry Plum where the horse seems to lose his self-control and attack whoever is nearest him, even without apparent provocation.

∩ Vine where the horse is persistently attacking another horse and you feel that he is trying to assert his dominance. But Larch may also apply, because the need to assert dominance over and over is a sign of fundamental insecurity.

∩ Beech where the horse cannot seem to tolerate the presence of another horse, and always lashes out when he is there. Genuine aggression during grooming can also be a Beech state – but ask the vet to rule out pain as a cause.

∩ Try Impatiens for flashes of temper that go as quickly as they come, especially if the trigger is a delay of some kind, such as not grooming or not providing food at the normal time.

∩ Walnut where the aggression follows a change of some sort, such as a change in owner or a new arrival in the barn.

∩ Red Chestnut or Chicory where aggression is shown by a dam towards horses and people who get too close to her foal. Red Chestnut is a fear remedy, and is appropriate where fear for the safely of the foal accounts for aggressive behaviour. With pure Chicory there is no fear, only a desire to keep the foal to herself.

Bud

Bud was born as one of a set of twins. The birth of twins is a rare event in horses, and when it does happen there are usually problems. This time was no exception. Bud's sibling died immediately after being born and their mother died a couple of days later. Bud's owner at the time had no option but to rear him by hand.

Bud's emotional problems began to manifest themselves when he started to nudge and nip his owner, the person who had hand-reared him. A young horse often does this kind of thing, but quickly learns from his mother's body language or from simple retaliation how much he can get away with. In the same way that we socialise our own children to human society, so mares socialise theirs to equine society. But Bud clearly did not understand that what he was doing was not acceptable. His owner did not know how to send signals he could read, and Bud did not know how to read the signals that she could send.

Things got worse when Bud started to chase people who came into his field. The owner tried to deter this by chasing him right back, but this turned out to be counter-productive. Bud became scared of humans, but still tried to come in close and nip them whenever he could. So the people mucking out his field started waving spades and forks at him so as to keep him away. Their show of aggression frightened Bud even more and he became openly fear aggressive. He began to bite. It was at this point that Bud's owner felt things were out of her control. She handed Bud

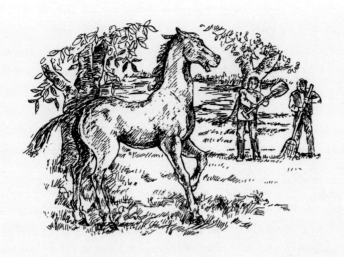

over to the UK Blue Cross organisation to see if they could help.

When he arrived, Bud showed many of the classic symptoms of chronic stress. He would lie in his stable for hours at a time. He was nervous around other horses, and herd members who had never been aggressive before tended to bully him. Consequently he spent much of his time alone. He had stress-related physical problems too, including diarrhoea and an unhealthy oily coat. And then his old habits started to come back. He began threatening staff mucking out his field. His handlers feared that things would soon escalate into an aggression problem similar to the one that his former owner had experienced.

The solution for Bud included a number of elements. One of the first steps was to find him a pair-bond. The staff chose a young Welsh pony, and Bud and the pony were removed from the main herd. This gave Bud the chance to get to know how to behave with other horses without the complex interactions of herd life. An aromatherapy shampoo was used to help deal with his seborrhoea. Finally, remedies were chosen to deal with the emotional side of his problems: Heather to help him be less insistent in his attempts at communication, so that he could listen better and learn that way; Star of Bethlehem for the shocks he had suffered from being the target (as he saw it) of aggression and bullying, and for the chronic stress he had lived under all his life; Wild Oat to help him find his true path in life and integrate with the herd rather than thinking he was half human; and Rock Water because he seemed to drive himself into repeating his behaviour, and needed to relax and accept himself for what he was. Later, Larch and Walnut were added to help his confidence levels and to assist the process of change.

Very soon after the new regime began Bud stopped being aggressive towards the staff. The aromatherapy shampoo brought about an enormous improvement in his skin. Best of all he began to pair-bond with the pony, which meant that the new couple were ready to integrate with other pairs and eventually with the full herd.

Bud's story illustrates the disastrous effect our good intentions can have. His original owner did her best when she raised him by hand, but the result for Bud was that he missed out on the chance to learn about horse behaviour from other horses. Ideally he should have had time with other mares and foals so that he could have learned horse manners, and learned that he was a horse.

Kinds of aggression: personal space

All horses need their own personal space, just like we do. Horses who are used to living in a group are careful not to invade each others' space uninvited. Instead they ask permission before coming near. The approaching horse uses a variety of communication signals to do this, the most obvious being the *way* he approaches. He moves deliberately and smoothly towards the other horse, then pauses at the first sign that his approach is not being encouraged. The horse being approached signals her feelings using looks and body position. A fixed look may be enough to make the approaching horse pause; a more obvious signal such as flattening the ears or turning her back may make him back off a little. By pausing or backing off, the approaching horse signals that he is not being aggressive. Gradually, if all goes well, he will be allowed to get nearer and nearer, backing off a little less each time, until he is finally allowed to enter her personal space.

Horses who have not socialised early enough or long enough with others sometimes don't understand the signals. Because of this they don't know how to approach other horses and feel confused when others approach them. They lack confidence, and because of this they will be more likely to make definite 'don't come closer' signals. In general, needing a lot of personal space is associated with a lack of confidence.

In a large field a horse lacking in confidence may be able to set his personal boundaries where he wants to, and so will not appear to lack confidence at all. The problem will show up only in situations where space is restricted, such as in a small paddock or while out on a hack with other horses. The latter can be an especial problem, in that the rider will expect to control how close he goes to the rest of the group. Under his rider's urging, the horse himself has no control over his personal space except to try to send stronger and stronger 'stay away' signals: stiffening his body, lifting and swishing his tail, lifting his head, generally looking aggressive. The other horses read the signals, but they too can't move away or pause as they normally would. Instead, they are ridden forward, and are sometimes urged to break unexpectedly into a canter in a manner that, to the anxious horse, could signal a clear threat.

If the situation continues, the horse lacking in confidence may take aggressive action to defend his space. He may end up kicking out at any horse who gets too close, which could of course be very serious for that animal. Even if he doesn't do this he will certainly be under continual stress, and will not enjoy the experience of being ridden.

A now discredited approach to this problem would be to force the insecure horse to ride in close company with others until he gave up signalling. But as we saw earlier, flooding actually makes fear worse, and the horse may begin to dread being ridden at all. It is far more effective and far less cruel to allow the horse to build up his confidence gradually. To do this, try to make the experience of hacking more fun for him. Ride him far enough away from other horses to let him relax. If he sends any 'stay away' signals at all, get the other riders to move their horses away further still. This mimics what would happen in the wild. You want him to complete an entire outing without once feeling under stress from the other horses. This will give his confidence a lift and he will look forward more to the next hack. Gradually you will find that he will be happy to have the other horses ride a little closer.

∩ The main remedy for lack of confidence is Larch, but this really relates to the horse's confidence in his ability to *do* things, such as jump an obstacle. The more likely remedy for lack of confidence in social situations is Mimulus.

Grief

Studies into the brains of horses have shown that their capacity to remember things is very similar to ours. The organisation of memory is the same as well. Some facts to do with what is happening now are stored in short-term memory, where they stay as long as they are needed but then fade. Other things go into long-term memory, which is where we and horses store the memories that create us as personalities: thoughts about our past experiences, where we live and have lived, and of course memories to do with friendships and attachments. We draw on long-term memory when we feel grief when someone we care about dies or moves away.

People who work closely with animals agree that they understand the concept of death, and that they mourn their dead.

The evidence for this is so strong that even experts who argue in general *against* the existence of animal emotions make an exception for grief. Naturalists have observed how elephants caress the bones of dead herd members, paying their last respects in stillness and silence, and in the case of horses researchers have been able to measure objective biochemical changes in their brains when they are separated from their pair-bonds. Horses can take months to recover from the loss of a pair-bond, displaying along the way all the familiar signs of loss of appetite and lack of interest in everyday activities. Even temporary absences can trigger mourning behaviour, because the absence may appear final to the horse. The remedies are a good way to start to help.

- Star of Bethlehem for the shock of separation and loss. This is an ingredient in Rescue™ Remedy, which is a good standby if you don't have Star of Bethlehem to hand.

- Walnut to help adjust to the change in surroundings or companionship. Try Honeysuckle instead if the horse is not trying to adjust at all and seems intent only on the past.

- Sweet Chestnut where a separation leads to hopelessness and complete despair. This would be the horse who really is pining away.

- Mimulus for horses who react to loss by displaying fear. Where the anxiety seems to be based on concern for the welfare of the absent friend substitute Red Chestnut.

- Restless, unsettled behaviour, where the horse looks lost and unsure of himself, might be helped with a number of different remedies. You could start by considering Scleranthus, Cerato, Walnut, White Chestnut, Agrimony, Larch and Mimulus.

Kinds of grief: death of a pair-bond

'Everyone of us has sympathy with those in distress,' Dr Bach once wrote, 'because we have all been in distress ourselves at some time in our lives.' Having understood that horses feel distress when they lose a loved one, just like we do, we will want to give special support to any horse whose pair-bond is about to be put down. This is a traumatic time for us too, but for the dying horse's pair-bond it is even worse, and he has no idea what is happening. Our aim must be to make the event as peaceful and non-traumatic as we can, for all concerned. This will help him grieve and recover sooner without suffering lasting emotional stress.

Perhaps the most common mistake we can make in this context is to anticipate the separation and part the horses at once with the aim of helping the healthy horse get used to the idea. This does nothing to palliate his grief. On the contrary, it brings it forward unnecessarily and may make things worse. In many yards he will be able to smell, hear and even see the dying horse from his new quarters. The only possible reason for separating close companions is if the healthy horse would be in danger of infection from the dying horse.

We would recommend the opposite approach wherever possible. Allow the horses to stay together day and night. This allows the healthy horse to get used to the idea that his pair is ill or injured, and so may die. (Just because horses don't whimper when in pain this does not mean they can't communicate: they use body language and facial expressions to signal when they are unwell.)

What about the actual moment when the dying horse is euthanised? Should the horses be separated before this happens? Perhaps surprisingly, there is a good argument to be made for allowing them to remain together even at this traumatic time. The advantage of allowing a horse to witness his pair-bond's death is that he will feel more in control of what is happening. This is less stressful than being removed to another part of the yard and not knowing where his pair-bond is or what is going on. If you do let them stay together during euthanasia, then allow him to remain with the dead horse for a further hour or two afterwards. This is what would happen in the wild. As most human cultures recognise, sitting up with the body gives us time to grieve and begin to accept what has happened.

However, this is not a blanket recommendation. You need to consider the personality and past reactions of your individual horse before you decide what to do. If he is already nervous of vets or loud noises, then he may be traumatised further by witnessing his pair-bond's death and become even more frightened of them in the future. But if you choose to remove him from the scene to prevent this you should still allow him to come back afterwards and be with the body for a couple of hours, for the reasons already given.

After his pair-bond has died, your horse needs time to grieve and come to terms with what has happened. As a guide to what to do, think about your own needs during a bereavement. You would expect a period of quiet – so don't take him along to a competition or suddenly go on a long hack with a group of friends. Adding physical stress to the emotional stress he has already suffered could make him ill. You would expect others to be there for you – so stay with him when he feeds and grazes, and groom him more often than you would usually. If his routine includes

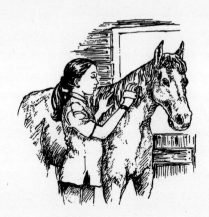

a daily hack, keep this up, but think of how far he would like to go rather than your own preferences.

Many horses continue to call for their dead pair-bonds for a time. This is quite normal. You can use the remedies or other complementary techniques to help him through this period. However, ask a vet or behaviourist to take a look at him if calling seems to go on for a long time or he seems unduly distressed.

If your horse lives in a herd then he may soon find a new companion with whom he can bond. But if all the other herd members are already pair-bonded and there are no suitable horses left you will need to help. After he has had a month or two to adjust to life without his dead companion, look out for a likely friend for him. The ideal would be a horse of the same sex, age and size. You should introduce the horses to each other slowly and carefully until they have pair-bonded. See the section called 'Meeting a new pair-bond' (page 160) for how to do this successfully.

Life experiences

Being born

New foals are far less helpless than human babies, and they mature fast. Within half an hour of being born they can be on their feet and feeding. Indeed, you should seek professional advice if a foal takes longer than two hours to stand, or longer than four to find the teat. It's essential that the foal gets his mother's milk before he is eight hours old, as the early milk contains antibodies that protect him against disease. After eight hours he will no longer be able to absorb them. If there are problems the vet may advise you to milk the dam yourself and feed by bottle. You should also call the vet if a foal has a fever or seems slow and sleepy or unaware of his surroundings. But a little shivering is normal at first as it helps the foal get warm.

Some practitioners believe that you can tell a lot about the personality of a foal even before he is born. Foals who move around a lot in the womb may be more assertive and demanding and end up as Vine, Impatiens, Vervain or Beech types. Quieter foals may turn out to be easy-going or retiring: Wild Rose, Agrimony, Centaury, Larch or Mimulus. Regardless of what type remedy you guess at, the remedies can help during the first few hours, alongside mother's care and the attentions of the vet where necessary.

- ∩ Walnut to help adjust to the new world, plus Star of Bethlehem if the birth has been traumatic in any way. These two remedies are often given at birth to human newborns as well.

- ∩ Olive if labour has been unusually prolonged and the new foal appears weak and exhausted.

- ∩ Hornbeam where the foal has had an easy birth but still seems slow to move, or Clematis for foals who seem barely alive or are sleepy. (But see the warning above about sleepy and slow-moving newborns.)

- ∩ Wild Rose or Clematis for foals who make no effort to seek out their mother.

- ∩ Impatiens for foals who seem unusually agitated.

Growing up

Foals are toothless at birth. Milk teeth start to appear after about ten days, and most young horses have a full set before they are nine months old. The second, adult set of teeth pushes through in subsequent years, the final teeth emerging when the horse is five or six years old. Teething foals may get irritable and lose their appetites in the same way that human children do. Sometimes they try to cool their mouths with water or earth.

Very young foals sleep a lot, just like human babies. The need to survive in the wild ensures that they soon take up more adult patterns of sleeping. At first they stick to a milk-only diet, but by about six weeks they will start to supplement this with pasture.

Young horses are curious and exuberant, like the young of most species. They enjoy playing and investigating new objects. Foals of both sexes very quickly do most of the things adults do, including grooming, running and communicating. As they grow they learn to interact with other horses by taking part in play-fighting. Colts will attempt to mount female horses, even their mothers, in practice for their later lives as full-grown stallions. The chief stallion will put up with this behaviour towards his harem for a time. If a three-year-old colt should try it on, however, he will soon be set to rights.

To be naturally comfortable with humans and other horses, foals need the company of both in the first two months of life, and ideally they should be habituated to the presence of humans in their first few days of life. To be really successful and avoid future handling problems, the process needs to continue right up to the point where the horse is first ridden. It is *not* good practice to turn the horse out with no human contact for three years and then suddenly back him.

As a minimum, a good socialisation routine would include:

- Handling the foal all over his body.
- Lifting all four feet.
- Approaching the foal from all sides and at different speeds and angles.
- Approaching the foal while carrying different objects, such as saddles, harnesses, lead ropes, grooming kit, etc.
- Leading the foal from both sides.
- Leading the foal into and out of horse boxes and trailers.

You should aim to make every interaction with the foal a pleasant experience for him. This way he will learn that he does not have to be afraid of humans.

Young horses shouldn't be ridden or worked too early. Breeders start working thoroughbreds when they are one year old, but most horses are allowed to wait until they are three or four. A longer wait is better, because working hard when they are not full-grown damages horses. This is why so many racehorses suffer from joint and leg problems.

At six years old a horse can be considered fully grown.

As for remedies, the following are often used during the first years of a horse's life.

- ∩ Mimulus for fearful foals, and for shy, timid horses who tend to get pushed around. Consider Centaury and Larch as well.

- ∩ Walnut to help adjust to teething and weaning.

- ∩ Chestnut Bud for foals who seem to take an especially long time learning social or feeding skills.

- ∩ Star of Bethlehem for anything that seems to come as a shock to the foal. This could include separation from his mother and the overenthusiastic attentions of human children.

- ∩ Rescue™ Remedy to get through any emergency in a calm frame of mind.

Weaning

Long-term studies into the psychological impact of separation in humans have shown that orphaned children can suffer from a life-long sense of bereavement following the sudden loss of their mothers. Clearly we can't simply assume that the same problems apply to foals and dams. Far less hard research exists. However, it would seem sensible to assume that similar types of creature placed in similar circumstances will react in similar ways.

The evidence we do have suggests that this is the case, and that abrupt and forcible separation is just as traumatic for equine mothers and their offspring as it is for humans. Despite this, horse breeders in the west have traditionally weaned foals when they are only five or six months old, parting them from their mothers all at once and taking elaborate precautions to keep them out of earshot of each other. The justification for this cruelty appears to be economic. Certainly it is not based on the nutritional needs of individual foals, many of whom would do better and turn out healthier if they suckled for longer. Nor is it done for good psychological reasons. Indeed, we scar foals for life by putting them through this experience, and make them more likely to develop severe emotional and behavioural problems. This is especially true when we remove them from their mothers and put them into solitary confinement in a stable. Horses denied

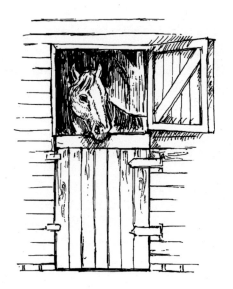

equine company early on lack social skills and do not know how to communicate effectively with other horses. As for the mares, their behaviour alone should tell us the anguish they go through. The sight of a mare throwing herself against the walls and desperately calling for her foal is not forgotten quickly. And professional breeders traumatise brood mares and put them through this agony on a regular basis, year after year.

In the wild, weaning commonly occurs when the foal is eight to ten months old, and happens gradually over a period of weeks. It takes place in the context of herd life, and is a positive step forward in life rather than the traumatic experience we see in our yards. Young horses enjoy short periods of independence at first, interspersed with adult reassurance. They learn how to behave from observing their mothers and the other herd members. They establish relationships with the rest of the herd before they leave their mothers for good, and can link up with a pair-bond and find their natural place in the herd pecking order. Often the stallion enforces the final loss of suckling privileges by driving the foal away when he and the mother are ready to mate again. But even then mother is still around, so that the event is less overwhelming. (If the stallion doesn't intervene the mother may continue to feed her foal for up to two years.) And always there is a clear social structure as a safety net. Fillies will remain in the herd along with their female relatives of all ages. Colts will join the bachelor herd after a short time in the nursery group.

How then can we give our own horses a more natural experience of weaning? The first step is to keep mare and foal in a field with other mares and foals. Over time the foals will take an interest in each other. They will play and interact more and spend correspondingly less time with their mothers. At the same time, and quite naturally, the mares will begin to reduce their supply of milk.

The second step comes when the foals are eight or nine months old. You need to put a temporary barrier across the field so as to separate them from their mothers. A piece of tape or a rope is fine – it will not injure any horse who runs into it and allows them to communicate with each other using their eyes and ears and body language. Just as a human mother feels more secure about her child's safety if she can see her, and the child feels happier if she can see mum, so the mare and foal will accept not being able to touch if they can still tell that all is well.

The first time you run a tape across the field the horses will probably run around for a bit or call to each other. This is part of the process, and can be compared to a child crying for a couple of minutes the first time mum drops her off at the nursery. If the horses quickly settle down and start to graze you can leave the barrier in place for a time. But take it away as soon as any horse shows continuing or persistent stress, and allow the two groups to get back together. The first session with the barrier may only last ten minutes and should not cause real distress to any of the horses.

Repeat this process over the subsequent weeks, gradually increasing the time the groups are separated until they can be apart for several hours at a time. When they accept this calmly you can move to the next stage, which is to separate the mares and foals into adjacent fields. Again, this allows them to stay within earshot of each other so that they know there is no danger. If this is managed well the two groups will begin to graze well away from the fence, and to set up their own separate grazing timetables. This is a sign of their growing independence.

For breeders, natural weaning is a more time-consuming process than simply pulling the foal and mother apart in one go. But the behavioural rewards are worth the effort. Mare and foal will be happier, more well-adjusted and easier to work with. This alone should convince any declared lover of horses that the natural way is the only acceptable way.

Rosie

The Blue Cross, a UK animal welfare organisation, took in Rosie after her owner lost his job and couldn't afford to keep her any more. When she arrived she was distraught, and sweating and shaking. The violent way in which she threw herself about told the Blue Cross staff that something was dreadfully wrong. On making enquiries they discovered that on that very day she had been separated without warning from her foal. As well as the usual anxiety at being in a strange place with strange people, she was having to face up to the immense grief and trauma of losing her foal.

Things got worse when the Blue Cross investigated further. Rosie had given birth before, and each time her babies had been taken from her without warning. We know that animals who suffer repeated trauma are less able to cope with their emotions, and in Rosie's case a series of abrupt and painful forced separations had left her severely traumatised. Her extreme behaviour showed that she was struggling to cope with her present bereavement, but in addition she had a lifetime of pain to deal with.

Eventually Rosie stopped throwing herself about. She was exhausted, but the pain remained. She began to show signs of severe depression, and would lie down in her field sleeping for hours at a time, looking for all the world as if she were dead. Staff could walk right up to her and get no response. She was kept outside 24 hours a day and had access to other horses, but she stayed by herself whenever she could. She was withdrawn, difficult to handle, and suffering as well from a form of stress-related asthma.

This was the stage things had reached when Rosie was first given Bach flower remedies. Her first mix contained five remedies: Star of Bethlehem for the shocks she had been through and for her continuing sense of grief and loss; Sweet Chestnut for her anguish and desperation, and the sense that she could find no way out of her pain; Walnut to help her adjust to what had happened to her, and to adjust better to her new surroundings; Centaury because she had a tendency to be pushed around by other horses; and Mimulus because of her continued anxiety especially when the other horses came near.

As well the remedies, Rosie was given behavioural help to get her used to other horses and gain in confidence. And aromatherapy was used to help her cope better with her fears and anxieties.

Within days Rosie began to improve. The staff at the equine centre found her easier to handle. For the first time she began to show an interest in the other horses, and in one other mare in particular, with whom she took the first step towards pair-bonding. She was still very anxious, however, so Aspen was added to the mix of remedies to help deal with what was starting to look like a general sense of anxiety.

Over the subsequent month Rosie established a firm pair-bond with the other mare. She became more settled with the other horses and established herself in the main herd. Eventually she was confident enough to act as a kind of babysitter for a younger laminitic pony. This involved being led away from her pair-bond and from the main herd and put in with the pony, who was kept apart because of the need to monitor his grazing. After a time she would return to her regular herd. She accepted all this without showing any distress, a sure sign of a well-balanced and confident horse.

Playing

Play is a serious business. Children playing trains together are learning to work as a team. Kittens pouncing on table tennis balls are practising their hunting skills. Puppies who wrestle each other are using skills they will use later on to assert their position in the pack. We are familiar with these forms of play because they take place in our homes, but other animals also play, including horses.

Behaviourists have calculated that as much as 75 per cent of all movements made by young horses are to do with play. They play with inanimate objects, with each other, and by themselves. This behaviour is innate: we see the first attempts at play in foals when they are only one day old, when they leap and skip around their mothers. Later they will practise galloping and tight turns, and work on their communication skills by pulling faces and waving their tails. When they are about a month old foals begin to play with other foals, and where possible will choose to play with others of their own sex. Colt play tends to be rowdier and rougher than that of fillies.

Horses who play together regularly are much better at reading each others' communication signals and for this reason get along better and adapt better to each others' moods. Games include play-fighting, which serves a similar function to the one it fulfils in dogs, and also gives the horse practice at facing up to a predator if one day he should be cornered and unable to get away. Chasing is a social game that strengthens relationships between pair-bonds and within the herd in general. In the game called chase and charge, the whole herd runs off in the same direction; this is play behaviour that humans have used to encourage horses to take part in races. Nip and shove involves two horses nipping each other about the head and neck and pushing against each other. If their necks overlap during this game the horses have established a close bond. In general, pair-bonds play together more often than other pairs of horses in the herd.

Among horses, injuries are rare because they play cooperatively. It would not be in the herd's interest for members to become injured during a play-fight. Other rules have been observed among playing horses. Play often starts in a relaxed moment with one horse signalling his desire to play by making playful movements. This causes the mood in the herd to change as other horses respond to the first. The weather is a factor in this, in that horses feel lethargic and are disinclined to play in hot weather. When play gets underway it tends to revolve around particular sequences or patterns that repeat with variations. It stops immediately if anything threatening happens.

Horses who live most of the time in stables can have difficulty with play. When they get together with other horses they lack the skills they need to join in appropriately. Play problems will often translate into problems with mating, since the social skills needed are similar. If they have been deprived of play opportunities for a long time they will overreact at the first glimpse of freedom. This, and not 'natural exuberance', explains the behaviour of the horse who bucks and runs wildly as soon as he is turned out into a field. Back in the stable, they will try to satisfy the need to play by playing with buckets, or in extreme cases by stereotypical behaviours like wind sucking and crib biting (see page 106).

Sometimes humans have problems with inappropriate play behaviour, as with horses who grab hold of the head collar when you try to put it on, or nip and shove you as you try to mount. From the horse's point of view, of course, these behaviours are not inappropriate at all. He wants to get your attention and enjoy a game. If you respond to his grip on the head collar by struggling to get it on or pulling it away from him then you are rewarding his behaviour by giving him the attention he wants, and with a game of tug-of-war to boot. To stop this kind of behaviour it is much better to completely ignore it. Give him attention in other ways, such as stroking him or giving him a box of toys, either before he sees the collar, or only after he has let go of it. The toy box can be especially effective, since all horses enjoy mouthing on things. Diverting his attention to things he *can* chew on is going to be more effective than taking away the only object within reach.

Inappropriate play behaviour should also be a cue that you may need to change his routine to give him appropriate outlets for normal play behaviour and for taking decisions and doing what he wants. Again, there is a parallel with the care of humans: providing opportunities to let off steam and take part in decision-making are essential parts of managing children, employees and horses.

∩ Enthusiastic horses who have trouble calming down could be helped with Vervain. This is also good for the frustration felt by a horse who wants to play but is denied the opportunity. (The long-term cure, however, is to give him the opportunity.)

∩ Agrimony is good for a horse who seems playful and light-hearted on the surface even when he is distressed and unhappy deep down.

Horses in season

Most mares are capable of breeding in their second year, but breeders tend to allow them to mature for a further year or two before having them covered. The breeding season runs from spring to autumn, and in this time mares will be in heat every two and a half to three weeks, each heat lasting about six days. Signs that a mare is in heat include a prominent vulva, irritability and constant tail-swishing. But the signs can be misread, and if the mare is not ready she will soon let everyone know by kicking out and biting.

Young colts can be wilful and may take expert handling. Adult stallions who only get to mate with a mare occasionally have a particular reputation for being especially temperamental, although the main cause of this is the behavioural restrictions placed on valuable stud horses, who are stabled most of the time and are expected to perform with the minimum of courtship. The practice among professional breeders is to use a less valuable stand-in stallion to test the mare's willingness to mate. If she stands still, passes water and raises her tail, this shows that she is receptive, and the understudy is led away and replaced by the star. This is extremely unnatural behaviour for a horse and will inevitably lead to behavioural problems.

Nobody is sure why, but some stallions are very particular about the coat colour of their harems and may refuse to perform with a mare of the wrong colour. One solution is to 'repaint' the mare by strapping a coloured blanket around her.

We would repeat the advice given in other sections of this book: think seriously before breeding horses. There is already an uncounted multitude of unwanted horses in the world. (See also the section on stallions on page 76.)

- Mares who get irritable in season and like to be left alone can by helped with Beech or Impatiens. The former is more likely where they resent changes to their routine, the latter where they seem impatient and in a hurry.

- Frustrated, tense stallions could benefit from Vervain or Impatiens. Vervain would be preferred for those that are especially wilful, although this could indicate Vine as well.

- Scleranthus can help sudden changes of mood.

- Mimulus is the remedy for known fear, which would include the stallion's fear of a flying female hoof.

- Loss of self-control generally could indicate Cherry Plum.

Pabla

Pabla was a three-year-old mare who had been selected for breeding. She had irregular seasons – at one stage she was always in season, but at the time she was seen she had not come into season for five months.

Pabla was subject to mood swings. One day she would be happy, the next depressed and cranky. She was very intelligent, confident and sensible, but tended to be highly strung when she got upset. Recently she had been under a lot of stress due to competitions, but she tended to get on with things as if nothing at all was wrong.

A number of remedies were selected, including Oak as a type remedy and Walnut to help her resist outside influences and not get upset so easily. But the main remedies were Scleranthus, chosen to help with her mood swings, and Mustard to help the depressions that seemed to come and go of their own accord.

Within a week the mare had settled down and was in season again.

Pregnancy

Once a mare has conceived she has to wait just over 11 months for the foal to appear. The gestation period is fairly flexible, however, and it isn't that unusual for mares to carry their baby long into the twelfth month. The first external signs of pregnancy come in the fifth month, when the pregnant bulge may start to appear, and a month later you may see the foal moving about. But a lot depends on the build of your horse. Bigger, bulkier mares may not seem to change that much. If in doubt ask the vet to do a visual examination followed by a blood test or scan to confirm the pregnancy.

You can ride a pregnant mare up to the sixth month of pregnancy, but you should avoid hard work and unnecessary excitement. After six months it is better not to ride at all. She'll need more food from the start of month nine. Feed manufacturers produce special feeds containing the right supplements. Daily exercise is important too, so be sure to turn out a stabled mare as usual every day and as much as possible. Most pregnancies pass off uneventfully, but problems can occur so consult a vet if you are worried. This especially applies if you notice any discharge from the vagina.

It is very rare for a mare to carry more than a single foal to full term. Mares who conceive twins often abort early on. Twins that do survive tend to be weak and immature.

- ∩ Walnut will help the mare adjust to the various changes she is going through.

- ∩ For tiredness caused by the physical strain of the pregnancy, give Olive.

- ∩ Try Hornbeam where the horse seem energetic enough when actually called on to do something, but is lethargic and slow at first.

- ∩ Mares who become especially lazy and show no interest in even the mildest exercise might be encouraged with Wild Rose.

Giving birth and after

A few weeks before she gives birth the mare's teats will enlarge. This is particularly obvious in mares who haven't foaled before. Then, towards the end of the eleventh month, the foal drops into the birthing position ready for labour to begin.

In the wild, giving birth is dangerous. The mare is completely helpless. No wonder then that the start of contractions is signalled by the symptoms of an increasing anxiety: sweating, restlessness, and the need to hide away. As a prey animal, there are obvious evolutionary advantages to giving birth in secret and in haste, and nature has given the vulnerable mother the ability to give birth quickly, and to choose when to give birth so as to avoid onlookers. Nine out of ten foals are born in the darkest part of the night, out of sight of all but the most vigilant of humans.

Contractions can go on for many hours. They increase in strength and frequency until the waters break. A few mares give birth standing up, but most lie down on their sides and stay that way for a time even after the birth. This allows blood to continue flowing down the umbilical cord and into the foal. Foals are usually born forefeet first. Most are born wrapped in a caul, a semi-transparent bag that breaks as the birth process completes. Soon after the foal has emerged, the mother stands up and grooms her baby by licking him. The umbilical cord usually snaps by itself as the mother gets to her feet. The new dam and her foal recover quickly. They can be back outside together the very next day.

Mares usually manage very well by themselves and do not need the help of anxious humans. Nevertheless you should call the vet for advice if labour is prolonged and fruitless or the horse seems to be in pain. One useful thing that you can do is to clear away any membranous matter that may stick to the foal's nostrils after birth and prevent him from breathing. And there are several remedies that might help during labour and immediately afterwards.

- ∩ Rescue™ Remedy to help keep mother and you calm.

- ∩ Olive where the mare seems worn out by the effort of giving birth.

- ∩ Oak to encourage a mare who has struggled on for a long time and needs some extra help.

- ∩ Hornbeam or Wild Rose, as appropriate, to encourage effort in a horse who does not seem to be trying very hard.

- ∩ Star of Bethlehem for shock.

- ∩ Walnut to help the mare adjust to the physical and emotional changes she is going through.

- ∩ Chicory or Beech if the dam seems unduly protective of the foal or intolerant of your presence.

Maria

Maria had recently had a foal. After the birth she turned very aggressive. She kicked out at her own foal and was hunting another mare and foal who shared her paddock. She always had a dominant nature but now she was uncontrollable and was risking hurting herself by running non-stop around the paddock.

Maria was given Cherry Plum for her loss of control and for the way she was hurting herself and her foal. Among the other remedies given were Vine as her type remedy, Beech to help her tolerate the other horses in the paddock, and Walnut to help her adjust to her new status of mother.

Within the week there were positive changes. She stopped running, and stopped attacking her foal, who was now able to approach her. She found it easier to tolerate the other horses in the paddock as well. She still displayed aggressiveness towards them, but no longer attacked. After two weeks she didn't need the remedies any more.

Life in a stable

We humans have to put in more work if we keep horses in stables. We must either muck them out once a day and change all the bedding, or use the 'deep litter' system and remove droppings and add fresh litter on an ongoing basis. We have to carry in all their food and water and keep them clean in the absence of opportunities for mutual grooming, scratching on trees and rolling in good clean dust. And we have to deal with the behavioural and emotional consequences of forcing animals to live such an unnatural lifestyle. Why do we do it?

Cost is one factor, because in some parts of the world owners think it is more expensive to keep horses outside. But the main reason is control. A trainer getting her horse ready for competitions wants to feed a carefully chosen diet that gives the maximum energy and the minimum excess weight all year round. She wants her horse to turn up at the show ring shiny and well groomed and not mud-spattered and dishevelled. Basically, then, stables are a convenience for people. We keep horses in stables because it gives us more control over what they do.

The average riding horse in the UK spends approximately 21 hours a day locked up in a stable, often alone and with little or no opportunity for social contact with other horses. The situation is much the same in most of mainland Europe. In America, Canada and Australia, horses are luckier and more likely to live in free-ranging herds. But even there horses being groomed for competitions tend to be put back into a stable, and around the world racehorses almost without exception are confined to stables for most of their lives. For a plains animal used to living in a herd this is extremely claustrophobic and disturbing. In addition, most stabled horses are only fed two or three times a day with perhaps a couple of hours' turn out. This severely restricts the horse's normal feeding behaviour – and grazing is second only to flight in terms of instinctive behaviour. We would condemn governments that imposed these kind of conditions on human criminals, yet riders, trainers and yard managers with decades of experience accept what we do to horses without comment.

We need to change the way we think about stables. A stable is a small box for keeping an animal in one place. The normal word for this kind of box is 'cage', and if we said and thought 'cage' instead of using the euphemism 'stable' we would have a truer picture of the world from our horses' point of view. This might lead us to look again at the whole tradition of stabling.

Already many zoos around the world have stopped putting animals in cages. The awakened consciences of keepers and the views of paying visitors have led to a revolution in the way zoo animals are cared for. Safari parks and landscaped enclosures are the new norm, and the old Victorian iron bars have been consigned to museums, where they belong. Few cat lovers or dog owners would allow their animals to be kept in cages. Some even refuse to visit animal rescue centres because they find the sights there too distressing. Horse lovers need to be as demanding over the welfare of their animals. The fact that distressed horses suffer in silence should not be a reason to let them go on suffering.

But is 'suffering' too strong a word? Isn't it just sentimental nonsense to say horses don't like living in stables? After all, carefully stabled horses have plenty to eat, permanent shelter from heat and cold, the best veterinary care, and appear physically well and able to cope with their work.

To find the answers to these questions, let's look at the science.

Researchers have identified specific areas in the horse's brain that monitor what is happening both in his body and in the external environment. These areas interact with each other, and when they do they are known collectively as the hypothalamus – pituitary – adrenocortical axis, or HPA for short. The HPA regulates the body's responses to internal and external events by releasing hormones. Different hormones are associated with different types of event. When something makes the horse afraid or stressed, or causes him pain, then the HPA will release a particular set of hormones. One of these is the adrenocorticotropic hormone. This enlarges the adrenal cortex and stimulates it to produce a steroid called cortisol.

Because we know about this mechanism, we can test urine or blood from a horse and have an objective measure of how stressed a horse is. If we find high levels of cortisol in a horse over a long period of time, this tells us, without any room for argument, that the horse is suffering from chronic stress. This is what researchers have done. They have taken blood samples from free-living and from stabled horse populations, and have tested their hormone levels. The tests show that horses in stables show much higher stress levels, while horses living at pasture are more relaxed. Behaviour patterns have also been analysed, and again stabled horses come off worse. The higher stress levels are reflected in the kind of stereotypical behaviour that we have already discussed in this book.

This research has been repeated and confirmed around the world. The results should be no surprise to us. Everything we know about how horses live when they have a choice – in herds, in the open, ranging across large areas – should prepare us for the idea that they will not find living alone in a small space and with little or no access to the open air a comfortable experience. The average hamster in a cage has *20 times more space* in relation to his size than the average stabled horse. And the hamsters most of us keep as pets prefer to live alone and underground...

What should you do if your horse is currently in a stable? In practice, there are many options open to you, depending on how far you are able to go to help your horse improve his standard of living. The important thing when considering the changes you can make is to bear in mind the horse's spatial needs (see page 73) and try to meet as many of them as you can. Here are some suggestions, in descending order of preference:

1. **Turn him out in a settled herd 24 hours a day.** This is the way horses live in the wild, and it is the best lifestyle for them. It meets all their spatial needs. As long as there is enough room for them to move at will and find natural shelter from sun and rain, almost all breeds will cope with most kinds of weather and do well. As a yardstick, the average British winter should not cause any problems.

2. **Turn him out in a herd for 12 hours a day, and bring the herd into an open barn at night.** Although not as good as the first option, this system does have the advantage of keeping pair-bonds and a stable herd together, although it isn't suitable for horses who do not already have a clear and settled social relationship. It provides additional shelter if your horses are especially delicate or the winter is especially harsh. The barn should be big enough to allow all the horses to walk around freely and feed on the hoof.

You shouldn't lock the horses up once they are inside, but instead give them access 24 hours a day to an open enclosed area so that they can move outside if the spatial pressures inside get too much.

3. **Turn him out in a herd for 12 hours a day, and enclose the herd in a field shelter at night.** The field shelter system is a variation on option two for horse owners who do not have a barn. It compromises some of the horse's social space requirements, but works well for older horses and for very delicate breeds, both of which feel the cold more than most.

4. **Turn him out in a herd or pair-bond for 12 hours a day, and enclose pair-bonds together at night in a shared stable.** Four ordinary stables can be converted into one large one by removing inside walls. This allows settled pair-bonds to remain together at night. Each member of the pair can relax more knowing that an extra pair of eyes are on watch. As well as this social improvement, the extra space means they can move around more.

5. **Turn him out for 12 hours a day and at night enclose in a yard with an unlocked stable.** Leaving the stable unlocked allows him to seek shelter if he needs it, but he can also stay outside – along with the other horses in the yard – provided they all know each other well.

6. **As option five, but nights out are taken in turn.** A less satisfactory arrangement than option five, but still a vast improvement on basic stabling, is to only allow one horse to roam free in the yard at night, and keep the others in. Even one night a week outside for each horse is better than nothing.

7. **Turn him out for 12 hours a day and at night have him**

in an unlocked stable with access to an open run. At one
Blue Cross animal shelter, cheap tape was used to create a
run for each stabled horse. At one stroke this trebled the
space available to the horse. It gave him the freedom to
exercise some control over his life without affecting the
other horses in the yard. An added feeling of control
reduces stress in itself. This system remains a big
compromise for the horse, who is still living alone, but at
least he can get out and see what is going on around him.

We will have made progress in our view of horses and their welfare
when we see option seven as a minimum acceptable standard. It
is a system that should be possible even in livery yards that will
not consider or can't achieve any of the other options. It doesn't
cost a lot of money, but it does have real benefits for the horse.
If your livery yard will not help you carry it through, and especially
if your horse is turned out for only a couple of hours a day, or
not at all, or is kept indoors all winter, then your job as a
responsible horse owner is to look for a better yard. Long term,
the kind of conditions he is living in will damage him
psychologically, and they may also lead to physical health
problems. The more we refuse to put up with unsuitable yards,
the fewer unsuitable yards there will be.

Life outdoors

As we saw in the last section the ideal way to manage horses is
in a herd and turned out as much as possible. Horses are social
animals and are inclined to get along with each other, but if your
horse isn't used to living in a herd and has spent most of his life
in stables then he may have problems adjusting to his new
conditions. You can ask your vet to refer you to a qualified
behaviourist if you don't feel you are in control of the situation.
But with care you will be able to manage most of the more

common problems. Here are some typical situations along with suggestions for what to do.

∩ **Your horse is bullying other herd members.** First, check that this is true aggression, consulting an expert if necessary. He might just be playing. If the aggression is genuine, it may be a dominance problem to do with finding his place in the herd, or it might be fear. (See page 119 for more on aggression.) Mimulus will help fear and shyness, and Walnut is good for all times of change, but at the same time you need to reintroduce him to the herd in a more managed way. Start by taping off a corner of the herd's field and putting the new horse in that section by himself. Leave him there for about six weeks, then extend the taped off area into a second corner. After a further two weeks, move a medium- to high-ranking horse away from the herd and into the taped area. Leave the two of them in this area for two or three weeks, or until they have pair-bonded, when you can begin to introduce the pair to the rest of the herd, slowing increasing the time they spend in the main field over a period of days.

∩ **Your horse is being bullied by herd members.** Assuming he isn't just playing, being bullied is often a sign that a horse has not learned how to get along with others, probably due to a lack of social contact when he was growing up. As with the previous problem, the solution is to 'promote' him to a secure position by pair-bonding him with a higher-status horse. Separate him from the herd and put him in an adjacent field. Introduce him over the fence to a high-ranked member of the herd. Only allow them in the same field together after they have begun to groom each other over the fence. After a further two or three weeks, when they have pair-bonded, reintroduce the pair back into the herd. Again take time to do this and increase their contact with the herd gradually.

⋂ **Your horse spends his day walking up and down the fence.** The likely reason for this is that he is feeling the absence of a pair-bond. If he has a pair-bond make sure they are turned out together every day. If he hasn't yet got one follow the steps given in the previous paragraph so as to find him a pair-bond and introduce them as a pair back into the herd.

⋂ **All the horses are chasing and kicking out at each other.** This means that the horses have not settled into a stable herd. Maybe they are turned out in different groups each day so that they don't form clear relationships with each other. The answer is to see that the same group goes out together every day. In a very short time a leader will emerge and pair-bonds will start to come together, so stabilising the herd.

If a herd isn't a possibility you may want to get your horse to share a field with another single horse. It's worth taking the trouble to do this well, because horses left in a field by themselves tend to become anxious and depressed. See the next section on meeting a new pair-bond for how to manage the introduction.

Some problems are peculiar to outdoor horses. Catching them can be difficult, for example, but as with everything else the answer is to look at things from the horse's point of view. Start by thinking about the way you approach him, and remember how another horse would do it. Don't march directly into his space, but approach indirectly and at an angle. Pause if he looks unsure, then keep coming.

Assuming your approach is not threatening, try to empathise with how he feels about being caught. What are the consequences for him? Are the things you do together fun for him, or only fun for you? Is everything you do together hard work? No sensible creature would want to be caught if it only ever led to shoeing, being hard-ridden and schooled, or 12 hours locked up in a stable.

If this rings a bell with you, the answer is to give him better reasons to associate you with fun and pleasure. Start by visiting him more frequently, and not only when you have some chore to do. Do different things when you are with him. You might stroke him and then leave, or put his halter on him but allow him to go on grazing while you take a walk around the field, or just stand next to him and talk or read a book. Try leading him out of the field to the yard and then feeding or grooming him there before taking him back and releasing him. Interact with the other horses in the herd as well, so he can see that they accept you. When you catch him give him a treat. Give another treat when you release him – this helps reinforce that being with you is a pleasant experience. (Food alone will not help you catch him, however. Wanting to stay outside and with his pair-bond will be a stronger desire unless he is especially hungry.) After a while he won't know what to expect when you come visiting, and if you are careful to make the most of your interaction with him fun he will start to think of you as being fun to be with. He will come looking for you when you arrive rather than you having to chase him.

When you are out and about with your horse the same rules apply. Try to make life in your company pleasant. Horses can become bored if they always hack the same route. Chop and change where you go, and take advantage of any ditches, hills, banks and streams that you come across to give him a new challenge. If the surroundings are safe enough, allow him to take the lead and find his own way home for a change – he will enjoy the stimulation of having something new to do.

In general, outdoor horses allowed to mix with others have far

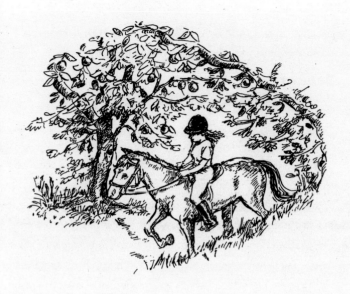

fewer emotional problems than solitary, stabled horses. They do have to deal with the weather, but a little preparation on your part can easily help. Wire boundaries don't provide good shelter in cold, windy weather, so choose a field with well-established hedges, trees and walls. Or build a shelter in the part of the field that the horses choose to stand at rest – they will show you which area has the fewest draughts and the best drainage. If possible, leave the shelter open on one side, facing away from the prevailing wind.

When other more personal problems arise the remedies can help you find a solution.

∩ Horses who are slow to make friends can be helped with Mimulus if they are shy or timid, or Water Violet if they seem reserved and slightly aloof.

∩ If a horse has been institutionalised in stalls and now lacks the confidence to explore more open surroundings, give Larch. Agoraphobia may need a mix of Aspen and Mimulus.

∩ Dominant animals who reject advances from new neighbours could benefit from Vine, Beech, Impatiens or Water Violet, depending on their natures.

∩ Walnut can help horses adjust to changes in living space and in relationships.

Meeting a new pair-bond

If you have bought a new horse in order to be a pair-bond for your current horse, then you need to manage the introduction well so as to get them to bond without either of them being a danger to the other. Start by releasing the new horse into a field next to the one occupied by your existing solitary horse. (If your current horse is not alone at all, but has a foal at foot, this is not a good time to introduce her to your new horse as she will be naturally inclined to chase the intruder away. Wait until the foal has been fully weaned.) Leave as soon as you have released the new horse, as normal greeting behaviour includes striking out with a foreleg, and you don't want to be in the way of such a vigorous handshake...

For a time the horses will watch each other. This allows each of them to get used to the other being inside his social space. Pausing is a way of asking for permission to get closer, so don't try to rush the process. Eventually they will move towards the fence to have a closer look. Once they are fairly close they will stay at an angle to avoid getting hurt if one of them strikes out with his foreleg. They will sniff at each others' nostrils in greeting, and after a few minutes will start exploring further by sniffing around the head and neck. During this time they stay tensed up, ready to move away at once if necessary. Signs of tension and interest include ear flicking and blowing, squealing and nickering.

You should leave the horses in their separate fields for at least a day or two. Signs that things are going well include the amount of time they spend nuzzling or grazing next to each other. If they start to groom over the fence this is especially good, because it means each has allowed the other into his personal space. Running along the fence together is another plus as this is recognised play behaviour.

Once you can see they are becoming friends you can move onto the next step. Lead the new horse into the existing horse's field and release him. As before, leave at once so as not to be caught up in the excited running around. Because you have been keeping your existing horse in a large safe field, there will be room for them to run around without danger, and enough space for them to keep apart if one of them feels nervous and needs to escape.

It's quite normal for one of the horses to start driving the other away or chasing him around. This may go on for a couple of hours at first, and then gradually tail off once the dominance relationship between them has been sorted out. If things don't settle down in a few days, and in particular if one of the horses becomes more threatening towards the other as time goes on, then go back to keeping them in adjacent fields and start again. Usually things do settle down, however, because horses want companions and so try to get along with each other. Try to separate horses as little as possible once they start to get along, and don't add other horses to the pair until the pair is well-established.

   ᴖ Walnut is good for all times of change and adjustment. You could add Walnut and Rescue™ Remedy to the water buckets of both animals during the process. The Rescue™ will help keep them calm during what is an exciting time for them.

Being sold

Look in the columns of the horse press and you will see column after column of ads offering horses for sale. You will see almost as many ads from former owners trying to trace horses they sold, sometimes years before. What does all this activity say to us?

If nothing else, it tells us that we buy and sell a lot of horses. The average horse in the UK will be sold six times in his life. Compare this with the normal lives of dogs and cats and other companion animals – they are thought of as unlucky if they go through more than one change of home. We wouldn't dream of selling the family dog if he got too old to chase rabbits, yet horses are swapped about like household appliances whenever we want a better model or the old one costs too much to repair.

But the ads tell us more. They tell us that some of us worry about the way we treat horses. That's why we place the 'lost' ads, and try to trace the whereabouts and welfare of animals we may not have seen for years. Usually our worries are based on the horse's physical welfare. Is he being fed well? What conditions is he living in? Do they keep him warm and pick out his feet properly? And of course we are right to think about these things. But the lengths some former owners go to suggest we might be aware of other causes for concern.

The two most important facts in a horse's emotional life are his herd and his pair-bond. Having these anchors in place helps him feel safe. He knows he can rely on the others to warn him of danger, help find grazing and water, and give him opportunities to play and practise his life skills. In the wild, fillies tend to stay in the same herds all their lives. Colts will move to a bachelor herd for a time, but even then they will be in a subset of their original family.

Each time we sell a horse and move him to a new home we shatter these relationships. The loss of his herd – the group of horses he knows in his current yard – is very traumatic. But the loss of his pair-bond is a bereavement for both horses. And we already know that horses feel grief and stress and shock, physically and emotionally, in exactly the same way we do.

What can we do about this?

There is no doubt that the best answer from the horse's perspective would be to stop selling them, and only take on horses if we can keep them for the 30 or 40 years that they are going to live. If this sounds idealistic it is probably no more so than the dreams of the first anti-slavery campaigners. Ways of treating fellow humans that seemed acceptable then are acknowledged now as unspeakably cruel and vicious. Perhaps in the future our 'common-sense' assumptions about animals will look just as wrong.

Having said that, if we feel unable to achieve perfection, that doesn't mean we should throw up our hands and accept the status quo. We can change things for the better by acknowledging and considering the horse's needs whenever we sell him or move him to a new yard. We can be advocates for his future well-being and make the kind of checks into potential owners that he would make if he could. We can give him psychological support. We can bear in mind that people and horses feel less distressed when they have some control over what is happening, and as far as possible ensure that he has some measure of control.

You can start the support process long before you actually sell your horse, by helping him be as well-adjusted and confident as he can be. Draw up a list of all the things that he is nervous of and plan to get him used to them, gradually and one at a time, while he is in familiar surroundings. If putting on a head collar frightens him or if he is scared of the vet, the same things will terrify him when he is in a strange place being handled by strangers. If he is not already expert at making friends with other horses, help him learn to communicate better. Take the time to introduce him to all the horses at his current yard. The more horses he meets now, the better he will cope with having to meet lots of new horses in his new home.

Once the sale process is underway, follow the lead of the better rescue centres and check on the suitability of prospective buyers. Don't sell him to the first person who answers your ad and comes to your yard. Instead find out where the buyer intends to keep the horse and go and check it out for yourself. You should be asking the buyer just as many questions as she asks you: How much turn out will he have? Will he be in a stable group? How many other horses are there? What prospects does he have of pair-bonding? The latter is especially important. If all the horses at the new yard have already paired up, your horse will be doubly alone. If possible you want him to be able to bond with a horse of the same sex and roughly the same age and strength as him: a three-year-old gelding and a 24-year-old arthritic mare may bond in time, but the situation will not be ideal for either of them. If you don't like the new yard and don't believe your horse will be happy there, don't sell him.

Before the sale is completed, get together with the buyer and between you come up with a list of things that she can do to help him settle in more quickly. This will be in her interest as well as the horse's. Look for things that he is familiar with in his current yard – toys, types of tack, his own rug – and for basic routines such as turn-out times, types of food and feeding methods. If the new owner can continue his current routine when he gets to the new yard, he will get comfort from already knowing some of the rules.

Finally, get the new owner's permission to check on the horse to see how he is settling in. If you offer this as willing help rather than an official inspection most new owners will be glad to accept. Make the first visit within a month of his moving, and the second about six months later. If you do spot any new problems that have developed since the move you will be able to help the new owner find solutions to them.

- ∩ Star of Bethlehem will help cope with the sense of loss following separation from his current herd and pair-bond. If he is severely affected add Sweet Chestnut as well.

- ∩ Walnut is good to ease change and help accustom him to his new environment.

- If he fails to thrive he could be homesick for his old yard: Honeysuckle is the remedy to choose.

- Changing homes is very frightening for horses. Mimulus for known fears and Aspen for general anxiety may both have a part to play while he settles in.

Rescue horses

Animals who have been mistreated in the past often need a lot of love and attention before they will respond to their new owners. The single most used remedy for rescue horses is Rescue™ Remedy. This has the advantage of being ready to hand, and it contains at least one or two remedies that will be useful to all traumatised horses. But with a little thought you can make a more focused choice and so be even more helpful.

- If a horse has been mistreated or has suffered past traumas, give Star of Bethlehem.

- If a horse is finding it hard to adjust to a change in circumstances or owner, give Walnut.

- If a horse is fearful of people or new situations, give Mimulus.

- Where fear is outright terror give Rock Rose, and where it seems general with no specific trigger try Aspen instead.

- Give Honeysuckle if the horse seems uninterested in his new life and repeats behaviour more appropriate to his former life.

Horses and competitions

From the ancient Mediterranean's addiction to chariot racing, through to thoroughbred horse-racing and rodeo events in the US, horses have long been used as a way for people to compete with each other. We may pretend that the horses are competing rather than us, but most experts agree that horses don't know or care if they win or lose races, although their ability to mirror the emotional moods around them means that they may well react to our feelings of success or failure. From the horse's point of view, competition is an exciting, if pointless, activity that puts him under a lot of nervous strain.

If you want to enter competitions, you and the horse need to practise a couple of times a week – any more risks boring the horse – in order to get used to what you have to do in the competition. Horses tend to associate places with particular activities, and if you only jump obstacles in the back field your horse might refuse at first to jump in a show ring. Build variety into training so that the idea of jumping – or running, or racing – is independent of place. And remember that too much training and competition can lead to burn-out for horses, just as it can for human athletes. They need a chance to rest and take part in fun activities so as to recharge their batteries.

Make sure your horse is used to his trailer, and to travelling, long before the day of your first competition. Ideally he should associate the trailer with nice, calm things like food and reassurance. He will not relax on the way to a show if all his journeys end with shouting crowds and stress. Horses know something is going on when their routine changes, so if you only ever arrive early and plait his tail on the morning of a show he will start to get excited or apprehensive right away. It can be useful to do some of these things on days off as well, then, so that the horse can stay relaxed a bit longer.

You should also get your horse used to being around other people and other horses. That way he won't lose his head the first time he arrives at a big competition. Finally, remember to use the remedies to help get your horse – and you – through the day with the minimum of angst.

∩ Horses who get nervous or upset at an event can be given Rescue™ Remedy.

∩ Give Vervain to lively animals who get overexcited and want to join in right away.

∩ If your horse tends to be too easy-going, or seems bored and lacklustre or inattentive, you could try Wild Rose or Clematis to help him become more interested in his surroundings.

∩ Horses who seem fearful or cowed can be helped with Mimulus.

∩ Consider Cherry Plum in addition to the type remedy for horses who lose their composure and lash out.

∩ Olive in the final feed of the day can help tired horses recuperate naturally.

More serious problems can arise if you have taken on an ex-competitor who has not been guided gently through competition. People often have trouble handling ex-racehorses in particular. Race yards are not the best places for horses to learn to like people. They often suffer from stereotypical behaviour because of their peculiarly stressful way of life. Typically, this has involved short, intensive exercise interspersed with hours locked away by themselves, concentrated feed and little or no turn out, and no chance to explore nor learn nor socialise with others. Often they actually fear people, associating us with unpleasant and confusing experiences. They have never had the opportunity (because they were too valuable) to learn that people can be fun or safe to be with.

If you do choose to adopt an ex-competitor, you can use behavioural techniques to communicate with him and gain his acceptance. Start by getting him to trust you personally and the new environment that he is in. Vary the things you do together, and make sure that they are mostly fun for him and at the worst neutral. Feed and groom him, take him in hand for a graze, go out on hacks to different places and give him the chance to look around when he gets there. His life as a competitor may have led him to associate some places or activities – like getting into a trailer or a tightened girth – with future stress. If so, try feeding or grooming him in association with the trigger so that he sees that there is no necessary link to something he doesn't like. A natural training system such as Parelli Natural Horsemanship will help him learn a new approach to working with humans. Make sure he has a pair-bond and that they (and preferably a whole settled herd) are turned out as much as possible.

When he trusts you completely, then you can start to introduce him to other human beings and – eventually – back to competition.

Accident and injury

If your horse has had an accident call the vet at once. Bach flower remedies do not treat physical complaints directly and can't mend a broken leg. What they can do is help your horse feel less sorry for himself while the leg gets better. This helps the physical complaint indirectly, because the immune system of emotionally balanced horses functions better, so they recover more quickly.

The remedies are one of the safest forms of treatment available. You can use them on your horse without having to worry that you will make things worse. Other forms of complementary medicine have more direct physical results, and in general you should only use them with the support of your vet and of a qualified practitioner in that field.

Injury

Even if we take extra care with our horses they are still more likely than their wild relations to have accidents and get injured. The blame for this lies with the unnatural things we ask them to do and with the artificial environments we put them in. We ask them to jump over obstacles that they could easily walk around. We put them in horse boxes and trailers and move them around so they suffer knocks to their legs and tails. We build barns and stables in vertical lines, with the result that they sometimes roll over

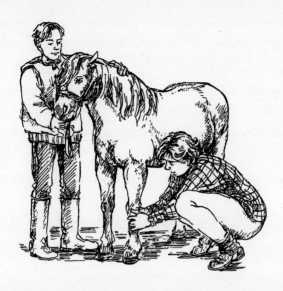

against a wall and can't get up again. Knowing all this, we need to be prepared, and have the remedies and the vet's number ready at hand whenever we need them.

- ∩ In all cases of injury or accident, reach for Rescue™ Remedy. For minor mishaps this will help your horse calm down and not become distressed. Where there might be an injury it will help while you seek veterinary attention – and you can take it yourself at the same time.

- ∩ Get veterinary help for all wounds. Do not try to remove objects such as thorns and glass from a wound yourself, since you may make things worse or leave fragments behind. The vet might advise you to clean daily with salt water, or tell you to use a hot compress to draw out any infection. If so, and following the vet's advice, you can add a few drops of Rescue™ Remedy and Crab Apple to the water. If the wound is in a hoof, it can be easier to add remedies to a basin of hand-hot water and have the horse stand the affected foot in it, but again seek the vet's advice first.

∩ You can apply Rescue™ Cream to minor wounds and scratches. With open wounds, avoid applying the cream directly. Instead you can apply it around the wound where it will help prevent leaking pus from damaging the surrounding areas.

∩ If there is severe and uncontrollable bleeding, try to press on the artery supplying the blood, or press down on the wound itself with a pad of some kind. Anything will do in an emergency, such as a towel or tee shirt or ice pack. Give Rescue™ Remedy by mouth, or apply it to lips and gums. Call the vet at once.

∩ Cover an injured horse with a blanket or rug – this will keep his body temperature up while you wait for help to arrive. Give Rescue™ Remedy or Star of Bethlehem to counteract shock.

∩ Horses who have been knocked over by a car should be kept still. Don't allow them to stand up in case of making any damage worse. Get immediate veterinary help and give Rescue™ Remedy.

Insect problems

A small percentage of horses are allergic to summer midge bites and react to the maddening itch by trying to scratch their manes and tails, pulling out hair and leaving bald patches on the skin and a tufted tail and mane. This condition is known as sweet itch.

Horses can also be allergic to bites from horseflies, which form hard lumps in the skin. And bites from red harvest mite larvae are a problem in stabled horses. The mites get into bedding and suck blood from the horse's legs causing a condition known as heel-bug.

- Ω Bathe sore, red areas around a sting or bite with cold water and Rescue™ Remedy.

- Ω Give Rescue™ Remedy by mouth to calm a frightened or distressed horse.

- Ω For sweet itch, try Cherry Plum and Crab Apple to counteract the out-of-control scratching. A proprietary insect repellent may help keep the midges at bay. Try to keep susceptible horses away from wetlands and inside on summer evenings.

Poisoning

Horses are sensible animals with a powerful sense of taste and smell and will not usually eat poisonous plants. But sometimes they do, and some acquire a taste for a particular plant despite its being dangerous. You may even be inadvertently feeding dried green bracken or ragwort to your horses in bundled hay.

The best cure for poisoning is prevention. Only use hay from a reputable source. Dig any poisonous plants out of your field before leaving horses in it to graze. Plants to look out for include the yellow-flowered weed ragwort, bracken, and of course deadly nightshade. Acorns and buttercups can be poisonous if your horse eats too many. Yew is extremely poisonous, as is laburnum, and mown grass soon ferments and goes toxic. This is why you should never feed garden waste to horses.

Poisoning is a serious matter for horses, as the way their palate is put together means that they can't vomit any noxious substances they consume.

- ∩ Seek veterinary advice at once.

- ∩ Give Rescue™ Remedy by mouth, or apply it to lips, gums and muzzle.

- ∩ Crab Apple is the cleansing remedy and may reduce the feeling of being poisoned. (It is not in itself an antidote to poison.)

- ∩ Horses poisoned with bracken may become excessively sleepy. Try giving Clematis in addition to any treatment recommended by the vet.

Burns

Burns can come from fire and from electrical and chemical sources. Horses do not usually suffer from burns, but stable fires are an ever-present danger to horses kept indoors.

If your horse suffers from a burn remember never to apply oil, butter or Rescue™ Cream to a hot area. The heat in the burn fries the oil or cream and causes more damage. Instead, cool the affected area by hosing with cold water. The sooner you do this the better. Add Rescue™ Remedy to the water and give by mouth (or rub it on gums, etc.) at the same time, so as to soothe the trauma and help your horse recover sooner from the stress. If the burn is anything more than very minor, or you suspect smoke inhalation or eye damage, seek the assistance of a veterinary surgeon as soon as possible.

Fever

Call the vet if you think your horse might have a fever. Warning signs include a dull coat and loss of appetite. The horse may defecate less or get constipation, so give plenty of greens and roughage, plus succulents like quartered apples and long slices of carrot to tempt him to eat. Keep a fevered horse warm, and if he is inside pile bedding good and high to keep draughts out.

○ Give Rescue™ Remedy or Star of Bethlehem at frequent intervals. The same remedies can be added to cold water and drinks or dropped onto ears, rubbed onto gums and so on.

○ You might give Hornbeam, Wild Rose, Gentian, Gorse, Clematis and other remedies to horses who are off their food, depending on how you read their current state of mind.

○ Impatiens can help to calm an agitated horse.

○ For lethargy consider Hornbeam, Olive and Wild Rose.

Shock

Signs of shock include a blue tinge to the gums and to the membranes around the eyes. The pulse rate may go up while body temperature drops. Horses can go into shock when they fall ill or have been injured, especially if there is internal bleeding.

○ Call the vet at once.

○ Use rugs, blankets, stable bandages, etc. to keep the horse as warm as possible.

○ Give Rescue™ Remedy or Star of Bethlehem.

Choking

Horses may choke if they feed on sugar beet that hasn't been soaked sufficiently, or on dry nuts or large pieces of hard fruit and vegetables – this is why you should always quarter apples and slice carrots lengthways before feeding them to horses. Symptoms of choking include drooling, regurgitation through the nostrils, and coughing and swallowing. Call the vet and try to massage the blockage to get it down. Only give water to a choking horse under veterinary advice because of the risk of getting liquid into the lungs.

Ω Give Rescue™ Remedy to keep the horse calm – and take it yourself while you wait for the vet to arrive.

Illness

On one level, illness is caused by bacteria and viruses, which is why you should get medical help to treat the physical agents of the disease. But despite the attentions of vets and grooms and endless supplies of food, water and supplements, wild horses catch fewer diseases and harbour fewer parasites than the average domestic horse. This is clear evidence that the lifestyle we impose on horses causes many of their ills. Bach flower remedies can help horses deal with stress and pressure, and the thought involved in using them helps you find out why your particular horse should have been the one who got sick.

For example, where there has been a change in the horse's life give Walnut to help him adjust. (The change might not be obvious to you. Maybe someone has taken a favourite toy away, or a favoured groom has changed jobs.) Consider too the way he is responding to the illness. A horse who follows you up the fence whinnying for attention is probably in a Chicory or Heather state. This state could actually be the underlying cause of the illness and not a symptom at all. Horses who mope in the corner feeling sorry for themselves will need Willow, while others who seem to give up hope need Gorse. Those who go about their round in a dogged, determined manner may well be ill because they have refused to rest. In this case give Oak.

We list here some suggestions for possible remedies, but they are only suggestions. Any of the 38 remedies could apply to your horse when he has a physical problem. You need to look at the horse, not the disease, when selecting remedies. And don't forget to take the remedies yourself so that you can be a better nurse – look again at page 68 for some suggestions. Finally, keep the Rescue™ Remedy handy for those emergencies where there is no time to think about how you and your horse feel.

- Cool sprains using bandages soaked in ice-cold water and Rescue™ Remedy. Dry the leg well afterwards to avoid cracking.

- Rescue™ Cream is good for many types of skin disorder. It's good practice to try a little on one area of the skin first, since some problems can respond badly to the application of any type of cream.

- Crab Apple is the cleansing remedy and will help any horse who feels contaminated or unclean.

- If the vet advises you to clean wounds or ears or eyes, etc., try adding a couple of drops of Crab Apple and Rescue™ Remedy to the water. (Never use neat remedies near the eyes.)

- Impatiens will help horses who become irritated and agitated when they are ill.

- Cherry Plum – where irritation or pain leads to the horse losing his self-possession and lashing out at you or biting or snatching at himself to the point of self-injury.

- Walnut may be useful where the problem is associated with a change in the horse's lifestyle or environment.

- Fear is a potent cause of stress in horses, and can lead to digestive upsets and many other disorders. Think about Mimulus, Aspen or Red Chestnut depending on the type of fear concerned.

- Horses who put themselves under stress might benefit from Impatiens, Vervain or Oak. Select the remedy that is closest to your horse's current state of mind: Impatiens for impatient types who want everything to happen five minutes ago; Vervain for enthusiasts who can't switch off; and Oak for horses who refuse to rest, struggling on at the same steady pace regardless of circumstances.

- ∩ Lack of appetite may be helped with Wild Rose, Clematis or Hornbeam – again, the right remedy depends on the individual horse.

- ∩ Choose Agrimony for horses who are obviously ill but remain playful.

- ∩ Choose from Wild Rose, Gentian and Gorse for animals who seem to give up when they are ill.

- ∩ Select Chicory or Heather for horses who become whiny when ill and demand attention.

- ∩ Try Willow for horses who retire to a favourite corner and mope.

Some horse illnesses are very serious and can prove fatal. Prompt action could save your horse's life, so always consult a vet if you think that your horse is unwell.

Fenster

Fenster was a seven-year-old who suffered from a leather allergy that left him red and sore where the bridle sat behind his ears, and where the rider's leg rested against his sides. He was a likeable character, very calm and reliable. Noise and upset never worried him and he never complained or lost his temper. Oak was selected as the type remedy, on the assumption that something must be wrong to cause the skin allergy but that he was not the sort to show it. This was given internally and some drops were also added to a base cream so that it could be applied directly onto the affected skin.

The Oak seemed to have some effect, in that his skin colour and hair condition improved, but after a time the improvement stopped. So Hornbeam was added – Fenster tended to be a bit slow to start – and within three or four weeks of using this mix all the hair had grown back and the leather allergy had gone. At the same time his reluctance to trot out faded and everything seemed less of an effort for him.

Old age

Old age in horses causes many of the same infirmities that it does in humans. Legs, joints and muscles stiffen as horses become subject to arthritis and rheumatism, wrinkles appear around the eyes, and grey hairs sprout around the muzzle. Dental problems are more frequent, hearing and eyesight fade, cataracts are more likely, and old horses feel the cold more than they used to. Even hardy ponies might welcome winter shelter in a barn for the first time.

Sometimes older horses show less tolerance towards foals and anything else that might disrupt their orderly lives. This may be due to the pain of arthritis, which makes the boisterousness play of youngsters harder to stand. On the plus side, however, older horses tend to be steadier than younger ones. Indeed, many parents prefer older ponies for their children on the principle that what the child doesn't know about riding the pony probably does. Most horses continue to welcome new experiences and variety, and can remain young well into old age if they lead an active life. Like people, they age faster when there is no stimulation. One of the sorriest sights in the horse world is a lonely old pony 'retired' to a solitary life in the furthest field.

- Try Beech for horses who are very set in their ways and get irritable when unexpected things happen.

- Walnut helps adjustment to difficult changes at any age, and is also good for easing your horse through the different stages of life.

- Try giving Olive or Hornbeam to horses who seem tired all the time.

∩ Try Wild Rose or Honeysuckle or Hornbeam for horses who lose their enthusiasm for life.

∩ Horses who cope well most of the time but seem to lose heart and confidence when things get too much for them could be helped with Elm.

∩ Oak is the remedy for those brave old plodders who keep going at the same even pace until they break down.

∩ General lack of attention to what is going on around them can be helped with Clematis or Honeysuckle.

∩ Horses losing their physical condition can get depressed. Try Crab Apple to help them accept themselves as they are.

Death

Horses can enjoy 30 or 40 years of life, but in the end death comes for us all. If your horse is lucky and you can afford good barn accommodation through the winter and the best veterinary care, then he may die old and healthy in his own good time. More often, sickness and increasing infirmity persuade owners to cut their horses' lives short to avoid suffering. In this case, the difficult choice is between having the horse put to sleep with an injection, or having him shot, usually with a special kind of bolt pistol strapped onto his head. The shooting option is the one chosen most often, perhaps because it can be seen to be instantaneous.

Having helped your horse's life with the remedies, you can ease his passing as well. And the remedies can also help your own grieving process, (and that of his surviving pair-bond – for which see page 130).

∩ Walnut can help a horse make the transition into death calmly. Rescue™ Remedy can also be helpful in keeping him calm.

∩ For yourself, try Star of Bethlehem for shock and for the sense of grief and loss.

∩ Take Clematis for the dazed bewilderment you may feel, to help anchor you in the present so that you can fully realise and accept the death.

∩ Select Sweet Chestnut when it feels that there is nothing left to live for and that the feeling will never go away.

∩ Take Holly for the desire to express anger by blaming someone and getting your own back.

∩ Walnut will help you adjust, or try Honeysuckle if you find yourself thinking in the past and losing concentration on the present.

From your point of view...

Horses and people

Our relationship with our horses is like every other relationship in our lives: we get back what we put in. Short-tempered and violent riders end up with reluctant horses who only do what they are forced to do – in other words, slaves. Most of the time slaves perform well, but they will rebel if they get the chance. On the other hand, if you ride with kindness and intelligence you can build a partnership with your horse. Far from rebelling when you do something wrong he will try to put things right because he is on your side.

Apart from any ethical considerations, then, there are good practical reasons for helping your horse have fun with what you want him to do. As a social animal he wants to cooperate. As a natural athlete he enjoys being fit and active. A sign of a true partnership is when his running and jumping give him as much pleasure as it gives you.

One way to help build a relationship with your horse is to groom him. Horses living wild groom each other to help keep their coats in good condition and stop them matting. The mane gets most attention because it has the longest hairs and so is the hardest area to keep clean. But beyond the purely physical need, grooming brings herd members together and helps the herd cohere as a unit. Riders who groom their horses can take advantage of this fact, and use the grooming session to emphasise to the horse the friendly relations that exist between them. It is even possible to mimic what horses do in the wild so as to underline the social meaning of grooming. So start by taking a sniff at your horse's nostrils – this is what his equine friends would do – then use your fingers to pinch at his mane. You won't be his friend if you try to get grooming over with as soon as possible – this would be like force-feeding your dinner guests and pushing them out of the door, then expecting a return invitation.

We also need to mind our manners when we approach our horses. As we have seen, horses have clearly defined concepts of space and are reluctant to let anyone get near without the due protocol being observed. If you are in a hurry to catch your horse in the morning and tear straight into the field waving a head collar, the horse is likely to interpret your agitation as cause for alarm and move away. You would get on much better by approaching indirectly and quietly, giving him time to acknowledge you and understand your peaceable intentions and invite you in closer.

Riding technique is often to blame for bad relationships. For example, inexperienced riders tend to hold the reins too tightly and pull on them to control the direction the horse goes in. A horse who is not sure of his footing needs to look down every so often to see that it is safe to go forward. If the pressure on his reins stops him from seeing where he is going he may refuse to go forward at all. With a little insight we can see his problem and allow for it in our riding. And we can go further still if we take the time to learn one of the natural riding systems that encourage communication between horse and rider, such as Parelli Natural Horsemanship.

When relations between horse and human break down it must be our job as leader to rebuild trust and confidence. This means taking a good look at where things are going wrong and taking kind and sensible steps to put them right. This can include using the remedies where appropriate.

- ∩ First, think about your own behaviour and take any remedies that you need to get your own approach back into balance.

- ∩ Give Mimulus to a horse who has been frightened by a human, or Rock Rose where the reaction is real terror.

- ∩ The same fear remedies are also good for horses who never learned to trust people when they were young. You might need to add Holly for the fundamental suspicion that sometimes accompanies fear in such animals.

- ∩ Cerato would be for horses who depend on humans to help them make decisions. They lack confidence in their judgement, and will look to their rider for confirmation before acting, as if checking that what they are going to do is acceptable.

- ∩ Heather is for horses who shamelessly seek out any and all human company, or use Chicory for equally demanding horses who restrict their attentions to their close friends.

- ∩ Vervain is for enthusiastic horses who get overexcited at the prospect of a hack.

Buying a horse
Choosing which horse to buy is one of the most important decisions

we make as horse owners. Because of this, most buyers ask vets to examine potential purchases before they buy, to see that the horse is fit and well and suitable for the type of use the new owner has in mind. For some reason, however, the checks often stop there. Few potential buyers take the next obvious step and check the horse over from a behavioural and emotional point of view. Yet if they did so they would avoid many serious problems. Physically your new horse can be the most talented in the country, but if you can't handle him, or if the farrier can't shoe him, or if he is bullying all the other horses in the yard, then the relationship between you will quickly deteriorate. Other horse owners may begin to resent his – and your – presence if his problems affect their horses. Your visits to the yard will become stressful instead of fun, as you turn up to firefight one incident after another. You may need to call in an expert to help resolve things, or you may end up doing what many owners do with problem horses: selling him on to somebody else or even having him put down.

To avoid these problems, or at least to know beforehand what the problems are going to be, you should take time to get to know a horse before you agree to take him on. This means assessing his personality. Qualified behaviourists use very exact scientific methods to do this, but for the purposes of assessing overall temperament a good approximation is usually good enough. You can learn the necessary methods relatively easily.

Carrying out a behaviour assessment means asking questions and seeing for yourself how the horse behaves in his current home. Visiting his yard once or twice is not going to give you enough contact time. Instead you should plan to visit five or six times before you sign on the dotted line. The questions you ask will be answered by the current owner, who should (if she has nothing to hide) be happy to help you find out all about the horse and his personality. (If she does refuse to help, our advice is not to deal with her.)

Your questions and observations will all be directed at finding out about five basic types of behaviour:

∩ How he behaves in the stable.

∩ How he behaves in strange environments.

∩ How he behaves with you.

∩ How he behaves with other people.

∩ How he behaves with other horses.

As you go through each category keep one overall question in mind: *how well is he coping with this?* Every time you ask this question, you will arrive at one of three answers: he may be relaxed, which means he is well able to cope; he may be mildly stressed; or he may be severely stressed. What 'mildly stressed' and 'severely stressed' mean can be defined scientifically, but for your purposes as a prospective buyer it's better to come up with your own personal definitions. So look at each of the five headings, and at the various activities measured under each heading, and decide before you start where you think 'mild' turns into 'severe'. The cut-off points you choose will reflect your own ability and willingness to deal with a particular problem.

For example, when you look at how he copes with being tied up, you might decide that a relaxed behaviour means standing still and patient while you get on with things. Mildly stressed for you might be when he lifts his head a little at first, but relaxes when you talk to him. Severely stressed might be when he pulls back as soon as you try to tie him.

The more times you define his behaviour as mildly or highly stressed, the more thought you need to give before you actually buy him. Be honest with yourself: can you cope with the challenge he represents, and will he be able to cope with the situation you intend to put him into? Problem horses can take up a lot of time and hard work and money.

Now we turn to our five headings. Under each one you will find questions to consider. Ask the current owner for her comments on each one. Then spend time with the horse to see for yourself how he behaves when he is in that situation.

◊ **How he behaves in the stable.**

- If he is stabled, does he exhibit any stable vices? Stable vices are a sign that he is clinically depressed due to the unnatural environment he has been forced to live in. You can rescue a depressed horse, but it will take work and commitment. As a minimum, you will need to keep him turned out all the time and find him a pair-bond. Can you afford to care for two horses?

◊ **How he behaves in strange environments.**

- Can he cope with being led away from the yard by himself? A frightened horse will seem especially anxious or try to get away and run home, or will not respond to commands because of his fear. The cause could be separation anxiety, or he may have been sensitised to being alone. In either case, you will have to work hard at counter-conditioning in order to teach him to be by himself. In most cases you will need professional help.

◊ **How he behaves with you.**

- Can you approach him? If he steps back or flattens his ears when you come close, this means he is nervous when humans get too close. His anxiety may well surface in other situations involving people. If he shows his teeth, this could indicate possible fear aggression.

- Can you put on his halter and tie him up easily? Horses that are not habituated to the halter or to being tied may raise their heads and clamp their tails to resist the halter and pull back when you try to tie them. This will be something you will have to teach him once you get him to his new home.

- Does the presence of other horses make it harder to catch him and lead him away? Sometimes horses are especially difficult to catch when they are with others because they do not want to be separated from their companions. Try approaching him with a head collar while he is with his herd to see what he does. Problems like this often get worse in a new home, and can require a lot of patience and professional help to overcome.

∩ **How he behaves with other people.**

- Do outsiders have trouble working with him? Be present when the vet arrives to carry out the usual physical checks and look at how the horse behaves with her. If he won't stand still and seems anxious as soon as she appears, then he may be sensitised to vets, which means he is so frightened that he may not respond to ordinary habituation techniques. Be there when the horse is shod to see how he is with the farrier. And keep an eye on how he interacts with stable hands, other riders, and so on.

∩ **How he behaves with other horses.**

- Is he well integrated with the rest of the herd? Look for quiet grazing in company with others. If he acts aggressively with the other horses (and if this isn't genuine play), then he may need help habituating to other horses.

- Does he have an existing pair-bond? If he and another horse spend most of their time together, grooming, grazing and playing, then splitting them may lead to separation anxiety.

- Does he seem anxious or ostracised? If other horses keep him away from the herd, this suggests he is not well socialised. This often means that he will be anxious in many situations, including interacting with humans.

- Does he behave well when ridden in a group? Fear can cause anxious horses to kick out at others, so try riding him in a group to see how he behaves.

(None of the above takes account of physical prowess and schooling. A horse's performance as a jumper or trail horse needs to be assessed separately by you and your trainer.)

We wouldn't want to suggest that you should never take on a horse with problems. You will find possible solutions to many of them in this book. You may have the skills, the patience and the resources to give even the most traumatised of horses a good home and a new start in life. But you do need to be prepared for the commitment and time involved. Going through the assessment processes here will give you a good idea of what you will have to cope with before you decide to make that commitment.

Adjusting your horse to a natural life

Throughout this book we have talked about the advantages of allowing your horse to live as natural a life as possible. To recap, here they are again.

∩ Advantages for the horse.

- The security of a pair-bond.
- Social contact with the herd.
- Freedom to feed normally.
- Freedom to move around, play and explore.

- Freedom from anxiety.
- Freedom from depression.

∩ Advantages for you.
- A calmer and more contented equine friend.
- Fewer 'aggression' problems.
- Fewer problems with routine tasks such as shoeing and visits from the vet.
- Less mucking out.
- No need to deal with stable vices.
- Money saved on bedding.
- A clear conscience.
- A richer relationship with your horse, based on mutual understanding.

Human beings have long believed that horses and other animals should be treated 'humanely', which means treating them in a reasonable way that does not cause unnecessary distress and suffering. True emotional healing for horses starts with understanding what distress and suffering mean to them. Having reached that understanding the next step must be to act on it.

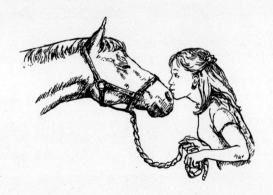

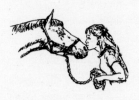

Part Three

Learning more

Other approaches to emotional healing

Many other therapies can help horses. Some are well known and widely available, such as orthodox veterinary care and chiropractic. But some of the less famous techniques are also worth exploring, especially as a combination of approaches often turns out to be more effective than any one in isolation.

Bach flower remedies are widely used by complementary therapists of various disciplines. Occasionally practitioners see them as a more appropriate alternative to their main therapy, but usually they are brought in as a helpful, complementary aid – the two therapies being used in tandem so as to approach a single problem from two directions at once. The remedies do not react or interfere with other treatments, which make them especially suitable to complementing other therapies in this way. (Note, however, that the alcohol preservative in the remedies may react with some medicines. Always dilute the remedies where possible, and consult your vet if in doubt.) Because the remedy drops can be given between therapy sessions, they are a good way of maintaining a sense of continuing progress.

We have not attempted to list all the possible approaches to emotional health that exist, or to give a full account of each therapy. Instead, what follows is an overview of some useful approaches, most of them like Bach flower remedies in that they approach health holistically. This means they take account of spiritual and emotional issues as well as physical symptoms. In general, these therapies work by stimulating a healthier and more vibrant flow of energy, and aim to restore harmony to the whole and reactivate the body's own healing resources. We have listed some good general guides to each therapy and/or a contact address so that you can find out more about it.

Acupuncture

An ancient Chinese medical technique, based on the Tao philosophy of yin/yang energy flow. In Tao philosophy, vital energy (chi or qi) flows along meridians, or energy pathways, in the body. This flow is either masculine, active and positive (yin), or feminine, passive and negative (yang). Ill health occurs if yin and yang are out of balance or the chi is blocked in some way. Treatment involves tapping into the flow of energy and dispelling the blockage. The energy within the meridian is stimulated and this in turn encourages a return of yin/yang balance and restored health. Traditional practitioners work by inserting fine needles into the skin at specific points, although some prefer to use heat or fingertip pressure.

Acupuncture should only ever be carried out by a qualified acupuncturist. If you feel it could help your horse ask your vet to refer you to a competent person with experience of treating horses.

> ∩ For more information see *Principles of Acupuncture* by Angela Hicks (Thorsons, London); or see the Other useful addresses section starting on page 202 for relevant organisations in the UK and the USA.

Aromatherapy

Aromatherapy uses the aromatic essential oils of plants. Different oils are indicated for different ailments and are used to restore both physical and emotional harmony. They are also used as an aid to relaxation.

Practitioners usually administer oils to horses by diluting them into a carrier oil and then massaging them into the skin or around the nostrils. In some special circumstances, they can be given orally, but this should only be done under the advice of a qualified aromatherapist. Many of the oils used in aromatherapy can be poisonous if taken internally.

Again, we advise you to contact a vet in the first instance for a referral to a qualified person who has experience in treating animals. You can treat your horse at home if you are careful, but never give essential oils by mouth or apply neat oils to the skin without consulting an expert. And remember that horses may lick oils off their skin if they can reach them.

∩ For more information see *The Art of Aromatherapy* by Robert Tisserand (The C.W. Daniel Co., Saffron Walden); or contact the Aromatherapy Organisations Council, 3 Latymer Close, Braybrooke, Market Harborough, Leicestershire LE16 8LN, UK.

Chinese herbalism

Like acupuncture, Chinese herbalism is an ancient medical system that goes back thousands of years. As with any holistic approach, it aims to treat both mind and body, and practitioners choose herbs constitutionally rather than for specific ailments.

The practitioner of Chinese herbalism uses a great variety of different herbs. Some, such as ginseng, are readily available and do not cause any unwanted effects, but others are harder to get hold of and may make things worse if you use them incorrectly. For this reason you should ask your vet to refer you to a practitioner in the first instance rather than try to pick the right herbs for your horse yourself.

> ∩ For more information see *Principles of Chinese Herbal Medicine* by John Hicks (Thorsons, London); or *Chinese Medicine – The Web that has no Weaver* by Ted Kaptchuk (Rider, London); or contact the Register of Chinese Herbal Medicine, PO Box 400, Wembley HA9 9NZ, UK.

Chiropractic

Chiropractic treats problems with the muscles and joints. Practitioners seek to adjust abnormalities in the musculo-skeletal system. This relieves pressure on nerves that could lead to many other forms of disease if left untreated.

As well as traditional chiropractic, some practitioners use a variant called McTimoney chiropractic. This uses a set of movements perfected by a well-known teacher and practitioner, John McTimoney. Practitioners of both forms of the therapy can treat animals, subject to referral from a vet.

> ∩ For more information on 'classical' chiropractic contact the British Chiropractic Association, 29 Whitley Street, Reading RG2 0EG, UK; for information on McTimoney chiropractic contact the McTimoney Chiropractic Association, 21 High Street, Eynsham, Oxfordshire OX8 1HE, UK; or see the Other useful addresses section starting on page 202 for relevant organisations in the USA.

Healing

Healing does not use pills or potions, but relies on simple contact between a healer's hands and the animal. It is based on the understanding that everything in life, whether physical matter or spiritual force, is a form of energy. Healing encourages the free flow of energy between the higher self – understood as the life force of the individual – and the individual's physical and emotional being. The healer uses herself as a channel, tapping into the spiritual energy of life and directing its flow to the individual being healed. Recipients may feel heat emanating from the hands of the healer, and a sense of peace and relaxation or relief from pain. Successive healing sessions aim to encourage a permanent return of this vital flow of energy, which in turn brings about an improved state of health.

∩ For more information contact the National Federation of Spiritual Healers, Old Manor Farm Studio, Church Street, Sunbury-on-Thames, Middlesex TW16 6RG, UK.

Herbal medicine

The use of medicinal herbs is thousands of years old. It reached its peak in the 16th century when Nicholas Culpeper wrote his famous book on herbalism, which is still in print today. Herbal medicines work by recreating balance within the body and are intended to be a treatment for the whole person, rather than for an isolated disease. They can be used as preventative as well as curative medicines.

You can take medicinal herbs in several different ways. You will find tablets, powders and liquid preparations in the shops, and dried herbs can be made into infusions similar to tea. Some herbal medicines have been prepared especially for the home treatment of horses and other domestic animals.

∩ For more information see *A Guide to Herbal Remedies* by Mark Evans (The C.W. Daniel Co., Saffron Walden); or *Complete Guide to Modern Herbalism* by Simon Mills (Thorsons, London); or contact the National Institute of Medical Herbalists, 56 Longbrook Street, Exeter, Devon EX4 6AH, UK; or see the Other useful

addresses section starting on page 202 for relevant
organisations in Australia.

Homoeopathy

Homoeopathy is the name of the system created by Samuel
Hahnemann, an 18th century German doctor. He found that a
very small dose of a substance known to produce certain symptoms
would help the body fight off a disease with the same symptoms.
This is known as the principle of 'like curing like'. For example,
the homoeopathic remedy Alium Cepa is indicated for colds that
cause running eyes and nose. It is made from onions, which in
their raw state will produce the symptoms the homoeopathic
preparation treats.

Homoeopathy uses the healing properties of plants, minerals and
animal products, all in minute doses. It treats the whole person,
and takes account of individual symptoms as well as personal
characteristics. Thus a homoeopathic remedy reflects the
constitution or personality of the recipient as well as the illness itself.

Homoeopathic medicines go through a process of potentisation,
which involves vigorous shaking between dilutions. This is called
succussion. The more stages of succussion a remedy goes through,
the more potent it becomes. This means that homoeopathic
medicines come in different strengths, the most usual being 6c
and 30c. You can buy 6c remedies over the counter, and you will
find preparations aimed specifically at horses and other animals.
There are also plenty of homoeopathically trained vets who offer
an alternative to orthodox medical care, even for serious illnesses.
To get in contact with one, go first to your own vet and ask for
a referral.

⋂ For more information see *Homoeopathy in Veterinary
Practice* by K.J. Biddis, *A Veterinary Materia Medica
and Clinical Repertory* by George Macleod, and
Horses: Homoeopathic Remedies by G. Macleod (all

The C.W. Daniel Co., Saffron Walden); or see the Other useful addresses section starting on page 202 for relevant organisations in the UK and the USA.

Osteopathy

Osteopathy is related to chiropractic – in fact the person who first developed chiropractic was a practising osteopath – and, like chiropractic, it involves manipulating the body in order to improve the functioning of its systems, tissues and organs. It is a holistic approach that focuses on the structure of the body, and treatment aims to bring about a return of vital energy and life force within the entire being.

In the UK, osteopaths are regulated by law under the General Osteopathic Council. Osteopathy is widely accepted by orthodox medical practitioners, and referrals to osteopaths are becoming more common. You will need to go to your vet first if you feel that your horse might benefit from this approach.

   ∩ For more information see the *Introductory Guide to Osteopathy* by Edward Triance (Thorsons, London); or contact the Osteopathy Information Service, PO Box 2074, Reading RG1 4YR, UK.

TTEAM and TTouch

TTEAM is the creation of a Canadian horsewoman called Linda Tellington-Jones. The initials stand for Tellington Touch Equine Awareness Method. This uses TTouch – a form of very light massage based on the Feldenkrais method – in conjunction with special exercises aiming to improve the physical and emotional balance of horses. TTEAM aims to teach the horse more about his own body and his movements, so increasing his self-confidence and inner balance.

   ∩ For more information see *Getting in Touch with Horses*

by Linda Tellington-Jones and Sybil Taylor (Kenilworth Press, Buckingham); or see the Other useful addresses section starting on page 202 for TTEAM's representatives in the UK or the USA.

Veterinary care

Natural therapies can provide excellent results, but most of them will not by themselves replace orthodox veterinary care. Registration with a vet is vital if you want to be sure that your horse is going to remain healthy and well. Your vet is a qualified medical physician who will be able to examine, diagnose and advise on the appropriate treatment for all kinds of condition. She will be able to perform blood tests, X-rays and scans to determine exactly what the problem is, and carry out surgery where that is necessary. Interventions like this may save your horse's life.

Vets are also well placed to refer you on to other practitioners who specialise in specific ways of treating animals. This may include referral to qualified complementary practitioners. Generally speaking, bona fide complementary practitioners will need to know that you have consulted a vet before they can begin treatment, and they will also want the vet to know about what they are doing. The different approaches of orthodox and holistic medicine, often diametrically opposed in their philosophy, can work together extremely well on a practical level. Make a friend of your vet, then. And if yours turns out to be entirely against complementary medicine you can always find another more sympathetic to your own outlook.

Suggestions for further reading

On Bach flower remedies

(The books listed here are all published by The C.W. Daniel Co.

unless stated otherwise. You can order them from your local book shop or direct from the Bach Centre – see page 201 for the address.)

◯ *Bach Flower Remedies for Animals* by Stefan Ball and Judy Howard – the most authoritative work on using the remedies to help animals, this can be used in conjunction with the present book. It explains the philosophical basis of using the remedies with animals and provides a guide to selection that can be applied to any type of animal. There are also dozens of genuine case histories to inspire you.

◯ *Emotional Healing for Cats* by Stefan Ball and Judy Howard – a companion to the present volume.

◯ *The Twelve Healers and Other Remedies* by Dr Edward Bach – Dr Bach's final word on his discovery explains in simple terms what the remedies are for.

◯ *Bach Flower Remedies Step by Step* by Judy Howard – a simple, general introduction to the remedies that provides all the information you need to start using them.

◯ *The Bach Remedies Workbook* by Stefan Ball – an interactive course that uses games, quizzes and other activities to teach the system.

◯ *Principles of Bach Flower Therapy* by Stefan Ball (Thorsons, 1999) – covers all the basic principles of the therapy, including how the healing process works.

◯ *Questions and Answers* by John Ramsell – the questions that are most commonly asked, answered by the world's leading authority on the remedies.

◯ *Handbook of the Bach Flower Remedies* by Phillip Chancellor – hundreds of case studies collected from early editions of the Bach Centre's newsletter.

- *Bach Flower Remedies for Women* by Judy Howard – covers all the major stages in a woman's life, with suggestions for using the remedies to help from cradle to grave.

- *Bach Flower Remedies for Men* by Stefan Ball – the companion volume to *Women* deals with everything from school exams to sex, work and retirement.

- *Growing Up with Bach Flower Remedies* by Judy Howard – how to select remedies for children of all ages.

- *Heal Thyself* by Dr Edward Bach – Dr Bach's philosophy of healing, told in his own words.

- *The Original Writings of Edward Bach* edited by John Ramsell and Judy Howard – a selection of Dr Bach's writings, some of them never published before.

- *The Medical Discoveries of Edward Bach, Physician* by Nora Weeks – the story of Dr Bach's working life, told by the woman who worked with him as he discovered and completed the system of flower remedies.

- *The Bach Flower Gardener* by Stefan Ball – how to use the remedies to help plants, illustrated with many real-life case studies.

On horses etc.

Writers on the subject of horses all have their own viewpoints and they don't always agree with each other. Some of the following may contain contradictory points of view, but they are all worth reading. Books with an asterisk after the title are particularly recommended.

- Budd, Jackie, *Reading the Horse's Mind*, Ringpress Books, 1996

∩ Hartley Edwards, Elwyn, *The Ultimate Horse Book*, Dorling Kindersley, 1991

∩ Johnson, Tricia, *The First-Time Horse and Pony Owner*, Pelham Books, 1989

∩ Lorenz, Konrad, *On Aggression*, Methuen, 1966

∩ May, Chris, *The Horse Care Manual*, Stanley Paul & Co., 1987

∩ Rees, Lucy, *Keeping a Pony*,* Swan Hill Press, 1995

∩ Roberts, Monty, *The Man Who Listens to Horses*,* Hutchinson, 1996

∩ Smythe, R.H., *The Mind of the Horse*, Castle Books, 1997

∩ Tellington-Jones, Linda and Taylor, Sybil, *Getting in Touch with Horses*, Kenilworth Press, 1995

∩ Vogel, Colin, *RSPCA Complete Horse Care Manual*,* Dorling Kindersley, 1995

∩ Wanless, Mary, *For the Good of the Horse*,* Kenilworth Press, 1997

∩ Waring, George, *Horse Behaviour: the behavioural traits and adaptations of domestic and wild horses, including ponies*,* Noyes Publications, 1983

Further study

The following are all available by mail order from the Bach Centre (see address on page 201).

∩ Cassette tape, *Getting to Know the Bach Flower Remedies* – side one gives you full descriptions of all 38 remedies, and side two gives you the chance to practise your knowledge in a series of exercises.

∩ Video, *The Light That Never Goes Out* – tells the story of Dr Bach's life and work.

∩ Video, *Bach Flower Remedies: a further understanding* – the trustees of the Bach Centre explain how to use the remedies.

∩ CD-rom, *The Original Flower Remedies of Dr Bach* – a useful self-teach tool that presents the indications for the remedies and instructions for their use alongside excerpts from Dr Bach's own writings and video clips from the Bach Centre.

You might want to attend a taught course that uses the remedies. Here is an overview of the different types on offer.

∩ *Bach Foundation-approved courses* are quality controlled by the Dr Edward Bach Foundation and run in many countries around the world. Courses are approved at three levels – level 1, level 2 and level 3 (practitioner training). The main course provider internationally is the Bach International Education Programme, but courses are also run by some universities and individuals. You can obtain more details from the Bach Centre. In the UK, there is a level 3 course of study that concentrates exclusively on helping animals with the remedies. Again, the Bach Centre can provide more information on this.

∩ *Correspondence courses* have a reputation for being overpriced and inaccurate, so be careful before parting with money. Any correspondence course that claims to equip you for professional practice should be treated with extreme caution. The Dr Edward Bach Foundation runs its own introductory correspondence course, recognised as equivalent to an approved level 1 course. Contact the Bach Centre for details.

◯ *Independent training* varies from short talks at local centres to full-scale courses costing hundreds of pounds. The quality and accuracy of teaching varies, so if possible look for a course run by a qualified registered practitioner. The Bach Centre may know of one near you.

Bach addresses

The Dr Edward Bach Centre

The Bach Centre is housed at Mount Vernon in the Victorian cottage that Dr Bach chose to be the centre for his work. The mother tinctures for genuine original Bach flower remedies are still made there today using the same methods that Dr Bach used. You can visit the house and garden and there is a shop on site selling remedies and educational material. Callers may obtain free help and advice by letter, phone or email.

The Bach Centre set up the Dr Edward Bach Foundation in 1991 with the aim of training and registering practitioners. The Bach Foundation approves training courses in many different parts of the world, including the USA, Canada, New Zealand, Spain, Brazil and Japan, and registers practitioners in 37 different countries.

Address: Mount Vernon, Bakers Lane, Sotwell,
Wallingford, Oxon OX10 0PZ, UK
Tel: +44 (0) 1491 834678
Fax: +44 (0) 1491 825022
Email: mail@bachcentre.com
WWW: http://www.bachcentre.com

A Nelson & Co Ltd/Bach Flower Remedies Ltd

You can contact Nelsons for information on local availability of genuine remedies anywhere in the world.

Address: Broadheath House, 83 Parkside,
London SW19 5LP, UK

Tel: +44 (0) 20 8780 4200
Fax: +44 (0) 20 8780 5871
WWW: http://www.nelsons.co.uk

Other useful addresses

Australia

ᴖ Blue Cross Society Inc, Lot 9 Homestead Road, Wonga Park, Victoria 3136. Tel: +61 3 9722 1265

ᴖ The Horse Protection Society of NSW, 103 Enmore Road, Enmore, NSW 2042. Tel: +61 2 9557 1011

ᴖ Humane Society of Australia (NSW), 1/75 Pittwater Rd, Manly, NSW 2095. Tel: +61 2 9977 6303

ᴖ National Herbalists Association of Australia, 287 Leith Street, Coorparoo, Queensland 4151

ᴖ Petcare Information and Advisory Service Australia Pty Ltd, Level 13, Como, 644 Chapel Street, South Yarra, Victoria 3141. WWW: www.petnet.com.au

ᴖ WSPA (World Society for the Protection of Animals) Australia, 46 Nicholson Street, St Leonards, NSW 2065. Tel: +61 2 9901 5205. Email: kmjones@ozemail.com.au

Canada

ᴖ WSPA (World Society for the Protection of Animals) Canada, 44 Victoria Street, Suite 1310, Toronto, Ontario M5C 1Y2. Tel: +1 416 369 0044. Email: wspacanada@compuserve.com

ᴖ World Wide Association of Equine Dentistry, PO Box 807, Turner Valley, Alberta T0L 2A0

New Zealand

∩ Humane Society of NZ Inc, PO Box 29-060,
Greenswoods Corner, Auckland 1003.
Tel: +64 9 630 0510

∩ RNZSPCA (Inc), PO Box 15-349, New Lynn, Auckland.
Tel: +64 9 827 6094

UK

∩ APACHE (The Association for the Promotion of Animal
Complementary Health Education), Archers Wood
Farm, Coppingford Road, Sawtry, Huntingdon,
Cambridgeshire PE17 5XT. Tel: 07050 244196.
Email: apache@avnet.co.uk.
WWW: www.avnet.co.uk/~apache/

∩ Association of British Veterinary Acupuncturists, East Park
Cottage, Handcross, Haywards Heath, Sussex RH17 6BD

∩ Blue Cross Equine Welfare Rehabilitation Centre,
Shilton Road, Burford, Oxfordshire OX18 4PF.
Tel: 01993 822454

∩ The Blue Cross Northiam Equine and Small Animal
Adoption Centre, St Francis Fields, Northiam, Sussex
TN31 6LP. Tel: 01797 252243

∩ British Association of Homoeopathic Veterinary
Surgeons, Chinham House, Stanford-in-the-Vale,
Faringdon, Oxfordshire SN7 8NQ. Tel: 01367 710324

∩ British Equine Veterinary Association, Hartham Park,
Corsham, Wiltshire SN13 0QB. Tel: 01249 715723

∩ British Holistic Veterinary Medicine Association,
The Croft, Tockwith Road, Long Marston,
North Yorkshire YO26 7PQ

- British Horse Society, The British Equestrian Centre, Stoneleigh Park, Kenilworth, Warwickshire CV8 2LR. Tel: 01203 696697

- The Farriers Registration Council, Sefton House, Adam Court, Newark Road, Peterborough PE1 5PP. Tel: 01733 319911

- Horses Protection, 17 Kings Road, Horsham, West Sussex, RH13 5PN. Tel: 01403 221900; helpline 01403 221927

- The Natural Animal Centre, Rushers Cross Farm, Tidebrook, Mayfield, East Sussex TN20 6PX. Tel: 01435 872556 (UK centre for Parelli Natural Horsemanship)

- Natural Animal Centre (Positive Horse Magic), Rushers Cross Farm, Mayfield, Sussex, TN20 6PX. Tel: 01435 872556

- RSPCA (Royal Society for the Prevention of Cruelty to Animals), Causeway, Horsham, West Sussex RH12 1HG. Tel: 01403 264181

- TTEAM UK, Sunnyside House, Stratton Audley Road, Fringford, Bicester, Oxfordshire OX6 9ED

- WSPA (World Society for the Protection of Animals), 2 Langley Lane, London SW8 1TJ. Tel: 020 7793 0540. Email: wspa@wspa.org.uk

USA

- Academy of Veterinary Homeopathy, 1283 Lincoln Street, Eugene, OR 97401

- American Holistic Veterinary Medical Association, 2214 Old Emmerton Road, Bel Air, MD 21015

∩ American Pet Association, PO Box 7172 Boulder, CO 80306-7172. Tel: +1 888 272 7387 or 800 APA PETS. Email: apa@apapets.com

∩ ASPCA (American Society for the Prevention of Cruelty to Animals, 424 East 92nd Street, New York, NY 10128-6804. Tel: +1 212 876 7700. URL: www.aspca.org

∩ American Veterinary Chiropractic Association, PO Box 249, Port Byron, IL 61275

∩ Humane Society of the United States, 2100 L St NW, Washington, DC 20037. URL: www.hsus.org

∩ International Association of Equine Dental Technicians, PO Box 6103, Wilmington, DE 19804

∩ International Veterinary Acupuncture Society, 2140 Conestoga Road, Chester Springs, PA 19425

∩ TTEAM, Animal Ambassadors International, PO Box 3793, Santa Fe, NM 87501

∩ WSPA (World Society for the Protection of Animals) USA, 29 Perkins Street, PO Box 190, Boston MA 02130. Tel: +1 617 522 7000. Email: wspa@world.std.com

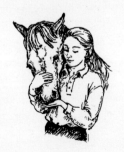

Index

abnormal behaviour, 87-9
  and see behavioural changes
acceptance, 128, 178
  and see resignation
accidents and emergencies, 33,
    51, 52, 168
  and see injury
acupuncture, 190
affection, 76, 118
  and see relationships with
  other horses, pair-bonds
aggression, 30, 40, 119-28
  and body language, 122-3
  and fear, 35, 110, 111, 120-1
  and food, 121, 122
  and grooming, 125
  and herds, 121-2
  and hyperactivity, 109
  of mares with foals, 120
  and personal safety, 123-4
  and see attacks on other
  animals, bullying, domination
agitation, 19, 48, 175
  and see restlessness
agoraphobia, 111, 159
Agrimony, 19-20, 65
  for
    grief, 131
    illness, 176
    owners, 69
    playfulness, 145
aimlessness, 48
aloofness, 47, 159
anger, 45, 179

and see frustration, irritability
anguish, 44, 101, 141-2
  and see anxiety, despair,
  distress, grief
anxiety, 20, 34-5, 40, 109-118,
    142
  and being sold, 165
  and grief, 131
  of owners, 70
  and stereotypical behaviour,
    109
  and see anguish, confidence
  lack of, distress, fear, grief,
  insecurity, restlessness
appearance, 26
appetite, lack of, 173, 176
  and see diet, food
approval, constantly seeking, 22
  and see attention seeking
aromatherapy, 191
Aspen, 20
  for
    abnormal behaviour, 89
    behavioural changes, 90
    being sold, 165
    illness, 175
    fear and anxiety, 111, 142
attacks on other animals, 23, 30
  and see aggression
attention seeking, 24-5, 28-9,
    174, 176, 181
  and see reassurance
avoidance behaviour, 34, 35